T0251222

The Student Guide to the Newborn Infant Physical Examination

This concise guide offers a comprehensive step-by-step framework for midwifery students to learn about all aspects of the newborn infant physical examination (NIPE), a screening assessment completed on all babies between 6 and 72 hours of age.

The Student Guide to the Newborn Infant Physical Examination encourages the reader to approach the examination in a system-based format, with case studies and practice tips to support learning.

The book offers:

- Evidence-based, well-illustrated assessment tools, which take into account the national screening committee standards, and is written by authors with both academic and clinical experience;
- A clear direction on how to perform the NIPE in practice while exploring the wider context of screening in healthcare today;
- Coverage of the changing role of the midwife, and the importance of understanding the whole context of the mother's care, health promotion and starting the practitioner-parent conversation.

The Student Guide to the Newborn Infant Physical Examination is a core text for all pre-registration midwifery students and a useful resource for qualified midwives, neonatal nurses and practice nurses.

Tracey Jones is a senior lecturer in Neonatal Education at the University of Manchester, UK.

The Student Guide to the Newborn Infant Physical Examination

Edited by Tracey Jones

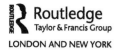

Routledge
Taylor & Francis Group

LONDON AND NEW YORK

First published 2020
by Routledge
2 Park Square, Milton Park, Abingdon, Oxon OX14 4RN

and by Routledge
52 Vanderbilt Avenue, New York, NY 10017

Routledge is an imprint of the Taylor & Francis Group, an informa business

© 2020 selection and editorial matter, Tracey Jones; individual
chapters, the contributors

The right of Tracey Jones to be identified as the author of the editorial
material, and of the authors for their individual chapters, has been
asserted in accordance with sections 77 and 78 of the Copyright,
Designs and Patents Act 1988.

All rights reserved. No part of this book may be reprinted or
reproduced or utilised in any form or by any electronic, mechanical,
or other means, now known or hereafter invented, including
photocopying and recording, or in any information storage or
retrieval system, without permission in writing from the publishers.

Trademark notice: Product or corporate names may be trademarks or
registered trademarks, and are used only for identification and
explanation without intent to infringe.

British Library Cataloguing-in-Publication Data
A catalogue record for this book is available from the British Library

Library of Congress Cataloging-in-Publication Data
A catalog record has been requested for this book

ISBN: 978-1-138-08638-8 (hbk)
ISBN: 978-1-138-08639-5 (pbk)
ISBN: 978-1-315-11101-8 (ebk)

Typeset in ITC Stone Serif
by Wearset Ltd, Boldon, Tyne and Wear

Printed and bound by CPI Group (UK) Ltd, Croydon, CR0 4YY

For my family, Andy my husband and my daughters Laura, Olivia and Madeline

Contents

Figures

Tables

Contributors

Natalie Anders qualified with a BSc in children's nursing before entering the specialism of neonatal care. There she gained several neonatal specialist qualifications such as the Qualification in specialty (QIS) and the enhancing neonatal nursing qualification, before completing an MSc in advanced neonatal nursing. She has experience working in a North West regional neonatal unit and now works as part of the North West transport team as an advanced neonatal nurse practitioner.

Melanie Carpenter is a registered midwife and an advanced neonatal nurse practitioner. She works as an expert witness for medicolegal cases and is a Care Quality Commission specialist adviser for neonatal care.

Dr Alison Cooke is a registered midwife, lecturer and researcher in midwifery, having completed a PhD in 2015. She has worked as a midwife in hospitals and the community, and then moved into a role working as a research midwife. During her PhD study Alison assessed the impact of topical oil use for infant skin care (the Oil in Baby Skin caRE study) and its effect on skin barrier function. Alison's research interests are infant skin care, advanced maternal age, maternal obesity and intrapartum care. Her overriding passion is to strive for improvement in maternal and fetal care and wellbeing, underpinned by the highest quality evidence.

Joanne Cookson is a midwifery/neonatal lecturer at Keele University, Staffordshire with an MA in medical ethics and law. She currently works for a neonatal network one day a week as a practice educator, alongside her role at the university where she teaches on both midwifery and neonatal programmes. Jo has a keen interest in the growing complexities of ethical debates that are witnessed within the neonatal intensive care unit environment.

Claire Evans has a role as the Antenatal and Newborn (ANNB) Screening Midwife at Warrington and Halton Hospitals NHS Foundation Trust, returning to the Trust from a 3-year secondment to Public Health England as a newborn infant physical examination (NIPE) implementation lead. During her secondment to Public Health England, Claire was the Project Lead for the Newborn Pulse Oximetry Screening Pilot.

Natalie Fairhurst is a trained paediatric nurse, who has worked in neonatal care for many years. She completed her MSc in Advanced Practice (Neonatal) in 2011, after which she began working as an advanced neonatal nurse practitioner at the Royal Bolton Hospital. Natalie has undertaken a study exploring parental involvement in decision-making in neonatal units, which will result in her being awarded her PhD in the coming months. She has recently moved to Sidra Medicine, a new state-of-the-art women's and children's hospital in Qatar.

Dr Jonathan Hurst is a consultant neonatologist responsible for newborn screening at Liverpool Women's Hospital. Jonathan has a significant interest in education, which includes delivering teaching as part of the NIPE course to undergraduate and postgraduate nursing, midwifery and medical professionals. He is also an examiner for the NIPE practitioner qualification from several institutions across the north-west.

Anne Lomax is a senior lecturer in the University of Central Lancashire where she works within the School of Community Health and Midwifery in the College of Health. Anne is currently Programme Leader for the MSc Midwifery course. For many years she has also provided the examination of the newborn module at post-registration and postgraduate level, predominantly for midwives both regionally and nationally. Anne is also a member of the NIPE UK Screening Committee Advisory Group for Public Health England and is involved in the development of national standards, competencies and learning resources for examination of the newborn. She has published several articles around the subject, and in 2011 edited the book *Examination of the Newborn: An Evidence Based Guide* for all practitioners involved in the newborn examination. In 2015, she produced a second edition of the text.

Christopher Lube is a qualified child health nurse who has spent a long career in neonatal care and NHS management before moving to work in governance. He is currently studying for his professional doctorate in health and social care focusing on governance and clinical accountability while working as head of governance and quality at the Liverpool Women's NHS Foundation Trust.

Carol Mashhadi is a registered nurse and midwife who has worked in academia since 2004. Carol joined the University of Central Lancashire in January 2017 as a senior lecturer and course leader for pre-registration midwifery. In September 2017 Carol was appointed as a principal lecturer and lead midwife for education, a strategic role that incorporates elements of leadership and quality assurance and maintenance of professional standards.

Sarah Paterson was appointed as an advanced physiotherapy practitioner specialising in development dysplasia of the hip and clubfoot in 2008. She works at the Royal Hospital for Sick Children in Edinburgh, where she leads the service for these specialities. She is involved in the teaching of medical staff of all grades with regard to hip dysplasia and clubfoot, and also contributes to the teaching on the Scottish Routine Examination of the Newborn course. She has travelled to Iowa, USA to study Ponseti's method for correction of clubfoot.

Michelle Scott qualified as a paediatric nurse in 2001 and has spent the majority of her career working in neonatology. She undertook an MSc in Advanced Clinical Practice at the University of Southampton in 2012, and has been working as an advanced neonatal nurse practitioner at University Hospital Coventry since. Michelle has recently been appointed as a senior lecturer at Coventry University, specialising in non-medical prescribing while also contributing to the delivery of the neonatal QIS course.

Kim Wilcock is a lecturer and admissions officer for the University of Manchester. Kim has worked as an academic across two Higher Education Institutions and has experience in course leadership, curriculum development and has held a position as Programme Leader for pre-registration midwifery. Kim has experience in obstetric emergencies, complex birth, simulation and teaching NIPE to Pre and Post Registration students.

Acknowledgements

I would like to acknowledge all those who helped peer review the chapters in this student guide; without their expertise and honest contribution this guide could not have been written.

I would also like to thank Timothy Walton from the University of Manchester for his support with Chapter 3.

I would specifically like to acknowledge the contribution made by my two artists. The illustrations for the book were completed by two young and enthusiastic artists, Jacob Gould and Finch Hartley, to whom I am most grateful.

I would like to thank those who gave permission to use images within this book.

Finally this book is dedicated to my family who have supported and coped without me throughout the writing process, which has been a long journey. And my Mum who always had faith in me. Thank you.

Introduction

Tracey Jones

The birth of a baby for any family is probably one of the most important life events. Every parent hopes for a safe and uneventful journey during this time. Approximately 750,000 babies are born each year in England, Scotland and Wales, and all of these babies will require a detailed 'top-to-toe' examination before 72 hours of age. This includes meticulous examination of the eyes and auscultation of the heart (National institute of Health and Care Excellence [NICE], 2006). This newborn infant physical examination is commonly referred to as the NIPE (pronounced nyp-ee) (Public Health England, 2018a). A second further physical examination is performed in the community to identify any abnormalities that may become detectable by 6–8 weeks of age, thereby reducing morbidity and mortality.

The NIPE differs from the comprehensive examination performed immediately after the birth, of which, as midwives, you may have a lot of experience. The NIPE screening is part of a national screening process whereby the content is specified by NICE (2015). This includes a holistic 'top-to-toe' physical examination of the newborn and a thorough examination of the eyes, heart, hips and testes (Public Health England, 2018a). More recently, the NIPE has increasingly been undertaken by midwives and neonatal nurses, due to reasons such as a decrease in junior doctors' hours, revisions in medical training and reconfiguration of neonatal services (Baker, 2010) and introduction of the working time directive (European Parliament, 2003; Clarke and Simms 2013). The Midwifery 2020 programme was commissioned in 2008 by the Chief Nursing officers for England, Wales, Northern Ireland and Scotland. The report underpins the vision of how midwives can lead and deliver care in a changing healthcare environment, reflecting policy and service direction. It also identifies the changes required to the way in which midwives work: their role, responsibilities, education and/or professional development to meet the vision. The report states that all newly qualified midwives will be expected to be proficient in examination of the newborn and expects curricular changes in the future, which has been an impetus for the increase in the NIPE being embedded into undergraduate education provision (Chief Nursing Officers of England, Northern Ireland, Scotland and Wales, 2010).

The examination at birth

During the examination after birth, the priorities are to highlight any immediate concerns or obvious signs of abnormality requiring the attention of a paediatrician and to facilitate an immediate medical review if required. For any practitioner to perform this examination competently and proficiently, and communicate any concerns to the medical team, they must have an understanding of newborn physiology and anatomy. It has been recognised that newborn anatomy and physiology theory content taught in undergraduate midwifery programmes differ immensely, so new opportunities for learning are constantly being developed to assist with understanding newborn management and care (Yearley et al., 2017). In 2017 NHS England aligned with other work programmes, such as Each Baby Counts (Royal College of Obstetricians and Gynaecologists) and Maternal, Newborn and Infant Clinical Outcome Review Programme (MBRRACE), to reduce avoidable term baby admissions to neonatal units; this work is known as the ATAIN project (NHS Improvement, 2016). This has been launched as a priority to avoid not only the unnecessary financial cost implications that accompany neonatal unit admission, but, more importantly, also the unnecessary separation of mother and baby. One key factor associated with the rising admission of term babies was the inability to recognise and manage simple neonatal conditions such as hypothermia or mild hypoglycaemia, highlighting a potential gap in knowledge.

Following the ATAIN project, NHS improvement launched a learning resource for practitioners working in the arena of newborn maternity services to educate re key areas linked to term admission such as hypothermia, respiratory complications and neonatal jaundice (NHS Improvement, 2016).

This resource examines the key areas linked to term admission to neonatal units, and offers educational resources to help recognition and action when a baby starts to deteriorate or presents with an abnormal presentation or observation. It is essential for any practitioner to have the knowledge and expertise to recognise any deviations from normal when carrying out any examination on the newborn; it is imperative that they should be suitably educated and competent. The examination of the newborn after birth has been part of a midwife's role for centuries and has offered reassurance to parents after the birth of their baby. In addition to this examination, midwives are required to undertake an assessment of wellbeing in accordance with Article 40 of the EU Directive for midwives 2005/36/EC (Nursing and Midwifery Council, 2009). The NIPE practitioner should be aware of the distinction between what is defined as the birth examination and what circumscribes the NIPE as a national screening programme.

Health screening

The formal examination of the newborn (NIPE) is a screening process that, in addition to the newborn midwifery examination, offers further detection and reassurance that there are no abnormalities present at the point of examination. We have come to recognise this further examination as the newborn infant physical examination or NIPE, although it has been referred to as the examination of the newborn (ENB). Medical screening takes place in many forms and you will be aware of some practices of screening that the mother will have encountered throughout her pregnancy. These are covered in more detail in Chapter 5 where you will be directed on how to assess the maternal antenatal history to help you understand why some interventions that may have taken place throughout the pregnancy might affect the outcome of the NIPE, and direct you to potential complications that might require referral.

The work completed by NHS England, the Department of Health, NICE and Public Health England exists to protect and improve the nation's health and wellbeing, and reduce health inequalities. Public Health England directs the national population screening programmes, which are implemented in the NHS on the advice of the UK National Screening Committee (UK NSC). The UK NSC makes independent, evidence-based recommendations to ministers in the four UK countries. The newborn hearing screen and the newborn blood spot test (Public Health England, 2017) are parts of the newborn screening that you could have encountered in practice and of which you may have some experience. Public Health England standards are based on ten themes that assess the whole screening pathway (Table 1.1).

This student guide focuses on the full newborn examination with specific reference to the NIPE screening, which facilitates early detection of congenital defects of the heart, hips, eyes and testes. The decision to focus on the four key points of the NIPE screen was the result of extensive work by Public Health England (2016). Current data show that around 1 in 200 babies may have a heart problem, 1 or 2 in 1000 babies may have hip problems that require treatment, about 2 or 3 in 10,000 babies have problems with their eyes that require treatment and about 1 in 100 baby boys have problems with their testes that require treatment. Any abnormalities detected or any clinical concerns identified will lead to a prompt referral for early clinical assessment by the relevant clinical expert (Public Health England, 2018a). This examination is an ideal opportunity to detect abnormality, make the appropriate referrals and, most importantly, offer reassurance to parents. It is imperative that the parents are involved in this examination and have been given information about the aim of the NIPE. After communication about the details and aims of the NIPE, the parents must give consent for it to be performed. There is additional literature available from Public Health England to give to parents, to ensure that they are clear about what the examination entails. Further information about imparting

Table I.1 The ten themes of the screening pathway
1 Identify population (to accurately identify the population to whom screening is offered)
2 Inform (to maximise informed choice across the screening pathway)
3 Coverage/uptake (to maximise uptake in the eligible population who are informed and wish to participate in the screening programme)
4 Test (to maximise accuracy of screening test from initial sample or examination to reporting the screening result)
5 Diagnose (to maximise accuracy of diagnostic test)
6 Intervention/treatment (to facilitate high-quality and timely intervention in those who wish to participate)
7 Outcome (to optimise individual and population health outcomes in the eligible population)
8 Minimising harm (to minimise potential harms in those screened and in the population)
9 Staff: education and training (to ensure that the screening pathway is provided by a trained and skilled workforce, with the capacity to deliver screening services as per service specification)
10 Commissioning/governance (to ensure effective commissioning and governance of the screening programme)

information and communication is found in Chapter 4. In addition to the four key areas of the NIPE, the baby is also given a full top-to-toe examination, the details of which are covered throughout the chapters of this book.

> ## CLINICAL TIP
>
> Ensure that you are clear about what leaflets are available in your department related to the NIPE and what training is available within your organisation related to gaining consent.

The standards for the NIPE have been developed to echo the screening programme themes (see Table 1.1), whereby a mandatory level of achievement must be recounted annually. Key performance indicators (KPIs) are used to continually monitor performance on key aspects of the NIPE, specifically how many babies are eligible and receive the NIPE screen and the timelines of this examination. These data are gathered and reported to local screening boards by key members of the team specified as screening lead professionals.

Public Health England (2018) standards recommend that all babies delivered in the United Kingdom are given a NIPE examination before they are 72 hours old and again at 6–8 weeks of age. The timelines of the examination are explored further in the text.

It is important that the parents are fully aware of the need for the further examination at 6–8 weeks of age, to assure them that this is a normal process and to avoid causing alarm or distress. The second check is necessary because the first examination cannot offer full assurance of cardiac normality, so based on evidence (McDougall et al., 2009), the further examination at 6–8 weeks has become part of the Public Health England (2018a) guidance. Examination of the heart is very important at this second check because it may be the first time that a murmur is audible. For example, if the baby has a ventricular septal defect (VSD), this may not have been apparent in the first 24 hours after birth (see Chapter 6B for further information and guidance related to the examination of the cardiovascular system).

The Public Health England (2018a) guidance recommends that the first NIPE should be carried out before the baby is 72 hours old; however, this is not always achievable in clinical practice for an array of reasons, and should therefore be completed as soon as is deemed possible. In addition to examination of the heart, hips, eyes and testes in boys, the practitioner also completes a top-to-toe examination of the baby, observing for any abnormalities. The other features of the examination are explored further in Chapter 6. Public Health England has published clear, easy-to-follow standards that can be used as guidance in relation to newborn screening (Public Health England, 2018b).

The decreasing length of stay for women after childbirth and earlier discharge have led to an increased requirement for more professionals to be qualified to complete the NIPE examination and an increased need for this examination to be completed in the community setting. This has led to a rising need for midwives and nurses to be suitably trained and qualified to carry out the NIPE. This student guide recognises the changes to education related to the NIPE and the chapters offer students a helping hand throughout that journey.

THINK POINT

Do you know who the lead professional is for the NIPE in your organisation?

It is useful to know this because they will be a point of information and resource both during and after your training.

Chapter 1: The newborn infant physical examination by Tracey Jones

Chapter 1 introduces you to the history of the newborn infant physical examination, and how this assessment has evolved over time to become not only a clinical screening tool, but also an opportunity to discuss any health promotion and parental concerns. This chapter uses evidence-based guidance to examine how the NIPE should be performed and why the focus is on the four key areas the heart, eyes, hips, and testes in boys. It helps you, as the student, to understand the complexities of the newborn examination in relation to the clinical evidence that directs national screening programmes.

Chapter 2: The development of NIPE roles in healthcare by Tracey Jones

Chapter 2 focuses on how the extended roles of the midwife and neonatal nurse have developed over recent years to include the NIPE. There is an exploration of the extrinsic and intrinsic need for practitioners to develop and progress within their role. This chapter covers extended roles in general, with a key focus on the areas of maternity and neonatal care to help the student understand why some undergraduate education has changed over recent years to include the NIPE. It includes 'think points' where students can consider their own experience of role extension.

Chapter 3: Communication skills in healthcare by Tracey Jones

Chapter 3 explores communication and explains why it is a key aspect of the NIPE. The practitioner not only needs to communicate with the parents during the examination, but must also have the ability to include the relevant detail when making a referral to an appropriate practitioner or service. Health promotion has become an integral part of the NIPE and has been shown to be a positive aspect of the reason why midwives are best placed to perform this screening process (Townsend et al., 2004). Continuity of care is also an important factor in midwives performing the NIPE. This chapter discusses continuity of care and identifies why women value this quality in their care provision.

Chapter 4: Maternal factors that influence fetal development by Carol Mashhadi

Chapter 4 considers the factors that might affect fetal development. This chapter explores the obstetric, medical, social and environmental factors that can be detrimental to fetal wellbeing. It assists you, as the NIPE practitioner, to recognise why maternal factors are influential and must be considered when performing the NIPE.

Chapter 5: Why the maternal history is important for the NIPE practitioner in performing a safe and thorough examination by Kim Wilcock

Chapter 5 directs the student how to assess the maternal antenatal history and understand why interventions that may have taken place throughout the pregnancy are relevant to the NIPE. Obtaining a detailed history from the woman on her general health, pregnancy and birth forms an essential component of the NIPE (Tappero and Honeyfield, 2010). It is vital to the NIPE that the practitioner has a clear history of any screening that has taken place and the results of this screening before embarking on the physical examination.

Chapter 6: The physical examination a step-by-step approach

Chapter 6 includes contributions from key specialists offering a comprehensive step-by-step approach to the NIPE. It offers guidance for the student related to all parts of the NIPE through a systematic approach, with think points throughout to enable knowledge checks to be completed. This is the largest chapter in the book.

6a: Examination of the head, including the ears, neck, eyes and neurological (tone) by Michelle Scott and Melanie Carpenter
6b: The cardiovascular examination of the newborn infant by Jonathon Hurst
6c: Examination of the respiratory system and chest by Michelle Scott
6d: Examination of the newborn abdomen and genitalia by Natalie Fairhurst
6e: The skeletal examination by Sarah Paterson
6f: Examination of the skin by Natalie Anders and Alison Cooke

Chapter 7: Congenital abnormalities by Joanne Cookson

Chapter 7 follows Chapter 6 with an examination of further abnormalities that might present on the physical examination. This chapter discusses the opportunity to recognise other deviations from the normal. It also discusses the short- and long-term implications of some congenital abnormalities.

Chapter 8: Overview of the NIPE and appropriate and timely referral pathways by Anne Lomax and Claire Evans

Chapter 8 offers a final overview of the whole NIPE; this chapter revisits the NIPE from start to finish and explores the process of referral. Referral is an important feature of the NIPE because some abnormalities require referral to a further service or specialty. This chapter assists the student to recognise what abnormalities require referrals and to whom they should be made. It requires the student to access some information from their employing trust to complete the learning opportunities included.

Chapter 9: Clinical competence and professional responsibility by Christopher Lube and Tracey Jones

Chapter 9 demonstrates why clinical competence and professional responsibility are important when taking on the NIPE role. This chapter examines the need for theoretical knowledge, clinical ability and accountability within healthcare, with reference to the Nursing Midwifery Council.

Chapter 10: The second examination in the community by Tracey Jones

Chapter 10 also explains the second examination performed at 6–8 weeks of age by the community practitioner. This chapter offers the NIPE student some knowledge to assist with parental discussion and reassurance.

The person carrying out the NIPE will be referred to as the NIPE practitioner throughout this book to recognise the growing number of both midwives and nurses and, in some organisations, other members of the unregistered workforce who are accessing NIPE education.

References

Baker, K. (2010). Midwives should perform the routine examination of the newborn. *British Medical Journal*, **18**: 416–21.

Chief Nursing Officers of England, Northern Ireland, Scotland and Wales (2010). Midwifery 2020: Delivering expectations. Available at: www.gov.uk/government/publications/midwifery-2020-delivering-expectations (accessed 25 April 2019).

Clarke, P. and Simms, M. (2013). Physical examination of the newborn: service provision and future planning. *British Journal of Midwifery*, August 16. Available at: https://doi.org.manchester.idm.oclc.org/10.12968/bjom.2012.20.8.546 (accessed 17 January 2018).

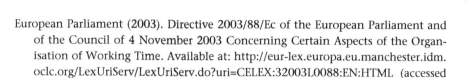

European Parliament (2003). Directive 2003/88/Ec of the European Parliament and of the Council of 4 November 2003 Concerning Certain Aspects of the Organisation of Working Time. Available at: http://eur-lex.europa.eu.manchester.idm. oclc.org/LexUriServ/LexUriServ.do?uri=CELEX:32003L0088:EN:HTML (accessed 16 July 2012).

McDougall, P., Drewett, R.F. and Hungin, A.P. (2009). The detection of early weight faltering at the 6–8-week check and its association with family factors, feeding and behavioural development. *Archives of the Diseases of Childhood*, **94**: 549–52.

National Institute for Health and Care Excellence (2006). *Routine Postnatal Care of Women and their Babies*. CG37. London: NICE.

National Institute for Health and Care Excellence (2015). Postnatal care up to 8 weeks after birth. Clinical guideline No 37. Available at: www.nice.org.uk/guidance/cg37 (accessed 25 September 2018).

NHS Improvement (2016). Reducing admission of full term babies to neonatal units. Available at: https://improvement.nhs.uk/resources/reducing-admission-full-term-babies-neonatal-units.

Nursing and Midwifery Council (2009). *Standards for Pre-registration Midwifery Education*. London: NMC.

Public Health England (2016). Newborn hearing screening programme: Standards. Available at: www.gov.uk/government/publications/newborn-hearing-screening-programme-quality-standards (accessed 17 January 2018).

Public Health England (2017). Standards for NHS newborn blood spot screening. Available at: www.gov.uk/government/publications/standards-for-nhs-newborn-blood-spot-screening (accessed 17 January 2018).

Public Health England (2018a). NHS Newborn Physical and Infant Examination Programme (NIPE): NIPE Programme Standards. London: Public Health England. Available from: www.gov.uk/government/publications/newborn-and-infant-physical-examination-screening-standards (last accessed May 2018).

Public Health England (2018b). NIPE Programme Standards. Available at: www.gov. uk/government/publications/newborn-and-infant-physical-examination-screening-standards.

Tappero, E.P. and Honeyfield, M.E. (2010). *Physical Assessment of the Newborn: A Comprehensive Approach to the Art of Physical Examination*, 4th edn. Petaluma, CA: NICU-INK Book Publishers.

Townsend, J., Wolke, D., Hayes, J. et al. (2004). Routine examination of the newborn: the EMREN study. Evaluation of an extension of the midwife role including a randomised controlled trial of appropriately trained midwives and paediatric senior house officers. *Health Technology Assessment*, **8**(14): iii–iv, ix–xi, 1–100.

Yearley, C., Rogers, C. and Jay, A. (2017). Including the newborn physical examination in the pre-registration midwifery curriculum: National survey. *British Journal of Midwifery*, **25**(1): 26–32.

Further resources

BAPM Newborn Early Warning Trigger and Track tool. Available at: www.bapm.org/resources/newborn-early-warning-trigger-track-newtt-framework-practice.

BLISS. It's Not a Game. Available at: www.bliss.org.uk/news/2015/its-not-a-game-a-year-on.

Lee, T., Skelton, R. and Skene, C. (2001). Routine neonatal examination: effectiveness of trainee paediatrician compared with advanced neonatal nurse practitioner *Archives of Disease in Childhood: Fetal and Neonatal*, **8**: F100–4.

Lomax, A. (2001). Expanding the midwife's role in examining the newborn. *British Journal of Midwifery*, **9**(2): 10–102.

MBRACE-UK Maternal, Newborn and Infant Clinical Outcome Review Programme (MNICORP). www.npeu.ox.ac.uk/mbrrace-uk.

Newborn and Infant Physical Examination e-learning: http://cpd.screening.nhs.uk/nipe-elearning.

NHS Screening Programmes newsletter. Screening matters. Available at: www.screening.nhs.uk/screening matters.

NHS England Reducing term admissions to NNU. Available at: www.e-lfh.org.uk/programmes/avoiding-term-admissions-into-neonatal-units.

NHS England Saving Babies Lives. Available at: www.england.nhs.uk/wp-content/uploads/2016/03/saving-babies-lives-car-bundl.pdf.

NIPE programme: http://newbornphysical.screening.nhs.uk.

Royal College of Obstetricians and Gynaecologists. Each Baby Counts. Available at: www.rcog.org.uk/en/guidelines-research-services/audit-quality-improvement/each-baby-counts/ebc-2015-report.

1 The newborn infant physical examination

Tracey Jones

Introduction

This chapter will help you to understand the background of how the newborn infant physical examination (NIPE) has become part of the midwifery and neonatal nursing, role and why there is a need for more practitioners to actively take on this extended role. The total number of births in England has fluctuated since declining to a low in 1977. In 2014 there were 664,543 births in England, compared with 566,735 in 2017. There were 679,106 live births in England and Wales in 2017, a decrease of 2.5% from 2016 and the lowest number of live births since 2006. In 2017, the total fertility rate (TFR) declined for the fifth consecutive year to 1.76 children per woman, from 1.81 in 2016 (Office for National Statistics (ONS), 2017). By 2020 the number of births will have increased by 3% to 691, 038, although by 2030 it will have begun to fall and is projected to be 686,142 (NHS England, 2016). Despite the fluctuations in birth rates all babies born in the UK are required to have a NIPE to confirm that the baby has made a successful adaptation to extrauterine life as part of the Public Health England screening; the aim of the NIPE is to:

> identify and refer all babies born with congenital abnormalities of the heart, hips, eyes or testes, where these are detectable, within 72 hours of birth.
>
> (Public Health England, 2018, Section 1)

This requires a significant number of skilled practitioners to be available. To understand why it is important for midwives and nurses to train to become NIPE practitioners, it is relevant to understand how the NIPE came about. The aim of this chapter is to explore the history of how the newborn physical examination has evolved over time to be recognised today as the NIPE.

The antenatal and newborn screening programmes should be seen as an integrated programme. It is important that the woman's journey through her pregnancy, birth and immediate postnatal period is regarded as a single, cohesive passage, and that information about mother, father and child is also incorporated, so that all the family history can be reviewed to avoid any missed early intervention.

As part of the education of students embarking on the NIPE journey, it is important to recognise that all practitioners, whether midwives or neonatal nurses, must have an understanding of the importance of the maternal documentation and the information that can be gathered from it to enable that journey to be smooth (see Chapter 5). The reasons for newborn examination are, first, to offer reassurance to anxious parents who look to the professional caring for their infant to give them assurance that there are no concerns and that their baby is healthy. To successfully achieve this it is important to recognise the limitations of the examination and have a full understanding of its benefits. It is important to remember that the NIPE is a screening process whereby your aim as a practitioner is to highlight any abnormality that requires a referral and not to make a diagnosis.

Midwives have been successfully performing examinations of the term infant as an extended aspect of their role since the first post-qualifying course was established in 1995 (Michaelides, 1995). However, there have always been specific examinations that the midwife/nurse, in accordance with organisation guidance, does not have as part of their scope of practice. There are some examinations that should be carried out by a medical practitioner and this is explored later.

THINK POINT

Take a moment to consider what has changed in the arena of childbirth over the past decade

---

The changing arena of childbirth

To recognise why there has been an increase in the need for more midwives and nurses being trained to complete the NIPE, it is important also to examine how the arena of maternity services and social dynamics has evolved. The factors that influence childbirth have altered. The physical act of childbirth has not changed over the years, but other aspects that might influence both the safety and the risk of childbirth, such as where babies are born and how long women stay in hospital, have altered significantly. The increase in women accessing assisted reproductive technology for childbirth has exposed the NIPE practitioner to further considerations. Areas that might need to be explored when examining the maternal history include previous in vitro fertilisation (IVF) attempts and if the pregnancy was a multiple birth (Davies et al., 2017), and the increasing age demographic of mothers:

Fertility rates decreased for every age group in 2017, except for women aged 40 years and over, where the rate increased by 1.3% to 16.1 births per 1000 women in that age group, reaching the highest level since 1949.The average age of mothers in 2017 increased to 30.5 years, from 30.4 years in 2016 and 26.4 years in 1975.

(ONS, 2017)

All of these factors require consideration by the NIPE practitioner.

The NIPE is clearly guided in that it should be performed within 72 hours of birth to highlight any abnormality at the earliest possible stage (Public Health England, 2018). Considerations such as home delivery and a speedy discharge from the acute setting need to be contemplated not only for monitoring of completion of the NIPE and reporting of the key performance indicators, but also to ensure that skilled practitioners are available to carry out the examination.

In addition to the evolving speed of maternal discharge, there are other factors that the NIPE practitioner must consider such as the age demographic of women giving birth. Childbearing at an older age has risen considerably and is becoming more common (Fitzpatrick et al., 2016). With this alteration, there is an increase in the potential problems that the NIPE practitioner must consider as more women choose to have their babies later in life. There has been a steady increase in the average age of first-time mothers from 27.2 years in 1982 to 30.2 years in 2014 to 30.4 years in 2016, a factor clearly outlined as a consideration in the 'Better Births' document (NHS England, 2016) which suggests that as a service the NHS must consider the implications on the risk to these women. According to the ONS (2017) women aged 30–34 years currently have the highest fertility rate of any age group since 2004; before this, women aged 25–29 years had the highest fertility rate, indicating that women are progressively delaying childbearing to older ages. With this increase in age comes added health considerations, and as the NIPE practitioner it is important to have an understanding of any maternal factors that might influence the NIPE. It might be that the mother is anxious or unwell, Was there assisted conception? There might be added pressures for the family or additional maternal medical conditions to consider. By examining the maternal notes in depth before embarking on the examination, this offers additional preparation, before the start of the communication process (NHS England, 2016; see also Chapter 5).

In addition to the consideration of the increased age demographic of women giving birth in the UK it is also important to recognise teenage pregnancy. Teenage pregnancies are continuing to fall and are currently at their lowest since the data first started to be gathered (ONC, 2017); however, there are certain parts of the country where this continues to be a significant consideration so it might be that you work within an area where there is a high number of teenage births. Baston and Durward (2017) highlight that teenage pregnancies have a probable rate of increasing due to the rapid age of maturity in young women, resulting in the first sexual encounter happening at a younger age. It is important for the NIPE practitioner not to make assumptions that all teenage births are a mistake; it is important that communication is a priority and that time is made available for discussion. Every mother will have her specific needs and it is important to be able to communicate effectively to ensure that full understanding of the NIPE has been made before consent is given. Public Health England (2017) clearly document in their standards for newborn infant physical examination that obtaining consent for screening is a professional obligation and a matter of respect between health professionals and the parent. The NIPE practitioner carrying out the screening is ultimately responsible for ensuring that the parent has an understanding of the examination and has given verbal consent. The decision to agree or decline the offer of NIPE screening should be clearly documented by the NIPE practitioner. As the NIPE practitioner, you will be required to verbalise to the parents any referrals being made and to ensure that all questions have been answered appropriately; this is in further depth in Chapter 3. There may be occasions when parents do not fully understand this information and refuse the examination. In this event first it is important to understand why this is the case. Do they understand what the aim of the NIPE is? Do they understand how the examination is carried out? If, after further discussion, the parents still refuse the examination and consent is declined, then it is important to be clear about your trust's policy because it might be that this situation requires you to seek support from a more senior colleague. Later in the book you will learn more about data monitoring systems such as the NIPE Screening Management and Reporting Tool (SMART), if after, further discussion, the parents continue to refuse for their baby to have the NIPE, it is the responsibility of the NIPE practitioner to clearly document on the data monitoring system the reasons for refusal, and in some cases there may be a need for a written declaration signed by the parents.

CLINICAL TIP

Explore what your trust's NIPE guideline directs in the event that a parent refuses to give consent for the NIPE screening. Being aware of this process will prepare you in the event that in the future you are the lead professional involved in such a situation.

Data evidences that the birth rate in the UK is seen to be decreasing, although the admission rates to neonatal units are in fact increasing (Royal College of Paediatrics and Child Health, 2017). This highlights an increased need for neonatal nurses to be skilled in performing the NIPE, which is evident in the increase in neonatal nurses accessing NIPE education. The (NNAP, 2017) has continued to highlight that a large number of babies born at term are separated from their mothers due to admissions to neonatal care, so speedy discharge is just as important from a neonatal unit as it is from a postnatal ward. As a result of the increased admission rate to neonatal units, there have been resources and learning platforms made available for all practitioners caring for the newborn. These learning tools assist the practitioner to develop skills to recognise and manage compromised newborns with the aim of reducing the number of term infants admitted to neonatal units (see Further resources at the end of this chapter).

THINK POINT

Consider what you understand by the term 'health screening'?

Health screening

Health screening programmes are commissioned by NHS England, Public Health England and the Department of Health. Health screening is not just a test. A test on its own will not improve outcome. All components of a care pathway need to be in place for screening to be effective. The key steps are:

- Identifying the individuals eligible for screening
- Inviting eligible individuals for screening
- Giving information and facilitating uptake
- Undertaking the screening test and making sure it is accurate
- Acting on screening results: referral, diagnosis, intervention and treatment
- Providing support and follow up
- Optimising health outcomes

(Public Health England, 2017)

The way the NHS approaches screening is constantly evolving as further evidence becomes available; embracing new technology offers the programmes further assurance. The pilot for the introduction of routine pulse oximetry has been completed by Public Health England and it is anticipated that this may be a recommendation as part of the cardiac examination because many trusts are actively including this as part of the NIPE; this is covered in depth in Chapter 6. The benefits of maternal antenatal ultrasound have increased the information that the NIPE practitioner can access before performing the examination, again offering further information to predate potential problems. This is an important note to make because practitioners can at times find themselves under pressure to complete the NIPE in a speedy manner. The reasons might be linked to assisting with faster discharges or succinct bed management; however, it is always important to review the maternal notes before performing the NIPE and that time is allocated and protected. Chapter 5 covers in detail some of the information that might be established from examination of the maternal history.

The NIPE role

THINK POINT

Consider why midwives and nurses have additional qualities to bring to the NIPE role. What other health-promotion strategies can be discussed with the parents during the allocated NIPE time?

The NIPE provides an opportunity for providing general health information, support and encouragement because this is often an interaction with parents when specific time has been allocated to that set of parents and baby. Jones (2014) suggests that the midwife, having influenced healthy choices in pregnancy, can now provide information relating to neonatal health during the examination. Feeding, nutrition, smoking, sudden infant death and immunisations can be openly discussed in this non-threatening environment, where mothers can be congratulated and praised at the same time as the NIPE is carried out. However, the challenges to maternity services are also well documented and it is no doubt that midwives can find themselves with heavy workloads (Royal College of Midwifery, 2016). Jones (2014) recognised that some practitioners have stated that lack of time and equipment and increased responsibility have been major barriers for performing the NIPE. Some services have recognised this and the importance of succinct NIPE completion, and have made the decision to allocate the NIPE role to a specific midwife or neonatal nurse on a shift-by-shift basis. This system can avoid the added pressures to both the busy midwifery team and the medical team who may also be covering the neonatal or paediatric units.

Whichever practitioner is allocated the role of the NIPE, examination of the maternal notes must be a priority. The notes must be studied before commencing the physical examination and busy workloads must not be used as a reason to overlook this important part of the NIPE. As a practitioner new to the role of NIPE, you might find yourself in situations in which you need the support of your more experienced colleagues, for example in the situation where the NIPE is refused. The communication to the parents of the importance of this screening process is imperative and is covered in more depth later in the book; however, a key point that you need to recognise is that the medical team should always be available for both referrals and advice. It may in some situations be that what should have been anticipated as a straightforward, nonmedical NIPE requires the input of a senior medical professional. The NIPE practitioner should always recognise that they are providing the NIPE, but referral to the medical team will be made when deviations occur or symptomatic risks are present.

There are certain babies who must have their NIPE completed by a member of the medical team because they may have additional medical needs that would require additional knowledge. Some of those might be babies born under 36+6 weeks' gestation or those who require admission to a neonatal intensive care unit (NICU), babies with a significant family history of genetic or congenital complications or who have had a suspected or confirmed abnormality at antenatal screening. It could be that your trust has highlighted that babies who have had a suspected trauma from birth, for example shoulder dystocia or Erb's palsy, require a member of the medical team to carry out the NIPE. It is important that you are clear about your local guidance and what babies you are allowed to examine; however, paediatricians should remain the lead professional where deviations from the norm are known or detected (Jones, 2014).

The systems used to monitor the NIPE have also been made more consistent, with the introduction of the NIPE SMART system in many trusts. It is important to remember that all newborn babies should have the NIPE performed within 72 hours, unless the baby dies or is too ill. In the case where the NIPE is missed, it is the responsibility of the birth hospital to undertake the NIPE unless the baby is transferred for specialist treatment to another hospital before the NIPE has been completed. In this case the receiving hospital would then be responsible. To audit the impact of this screening process, there must be an efficient process in place to document eligibility, completion, outcome and referrals. The NIPE SMART is such a system providing cohort management. NIPE SMART is an IT solution for the recording of the newborn examination of all babies residing in England (Public Health England, 2018). It provides a robust failsafe system and a consistent means of capturing data. This chapter has offered you the evidence in relation to key aspects of the NIPE and the influences that have led to the increase in more practitioners completing NIPE education. The focus on monitoring and role allocation has been the key point of this chapter which leads to further direction around the changing role of the practitioner caring for the newborn.

References

Baston, H. and Durward, H. (2017). *Examination of the Newborn: A practical guide*, 3rd edn. London: Routledge.

Davies, M.J., Rumbold, A.R., Marino, J.L., Willson, K., Giles, L., Whitrow, M.J. et al. (2017). Maternal factors and the risk of birth defects after IVF and ICSI: A whole of population cohort study. *British Journal of Obstetrics and Gynaecology*, **124**: 1537–44.

Fitzpatrick, K.E., Tuffnell, D., Kurinczuk, J.J. and Knight, M. (2016). Pregnancy at very advanced maternal age: A UK population-based cohort study. *British Journal of Obstetrics and Gynaecology*, **124**: 1097–106.

Jones, L. (2014). Examination of the newborn – medical or holistic screening tool? *MIDIRS Midwifery Digest*, **24**(1): 93–8.

Michaelides, S. (1995). A deeper knowledge. *Nursing Times*, **91**: 59–61.

NHS England (2016). Better National Maternity Review: Improving outcomes of maternity services in England. A five year forward view for maternity care. Available at: www.england.nhs.uk/mat-transformation/implementing-better-births/mat-review (accessed 1 September 2018).

Office for National Statistics (2017). Births in England and Wales: Statistical bulletin Available at: www.ons.gov.uk/peoplepopulationandcommunity/birthsdeaths andmarriages/livebirths/bulletins/birthsummarytablesenglandandwales/2017 (accessed 1 September 2018).

Public Health England (2017). NHS Screening Programmes: Newborn infant physical examination. Available at: https://cpdscreening.phe.org.uk/induction-resource/nipe (accessed 1 September 2018).

Royal College of Paediatrics and Child Health (2017). National Neonatal Audit Programme. Available at: www.rcpch.ac.uk/work-we-do/quality-improvement-patient-safety/national-neonatal-audit-programme-nnap (accessed 1 September 2018).

Royal College of Midwifery (2016). Why midwives leave – revisited October 2016. Available at: www.rcm.org.uk/sites/default/files/Why%20Midwives%20Leave%20Revisted%20-%20October%202016.pdf (accessed 1 September 2018).

Further resources

British Association of Perinatal Medicine (2015). Newborn Early Warning Trigger and Track (NEWTT): A Framework for Practice April. Available at: www.bapm.org/resources/newborn-early-warning-trigger-track-newtt-framework-practice (accessed 1 October 2018).

NHS Improvement (2017). Reducing harm leading to avoidable admission of full-term babies into neonatal units: Findings and resources for improvement, February. Available at: https://improvement.nhs.uk/resources/preventing-avoidable-admissionsfull-term-babies (accessed 1 October 2018).

2 The changing role of the practitioner caring for the newborn

Tracey Jones

Introduction

The NHS newborn infant physical examination (NIPE) is an established and integral element of child health surveillance in the UK, and is based on standards set by the UK National Screening Committee (Department of Health, 2008; Public Health England, 2018). This chapter aims to help you understand why you have been supported, either during your undergraduate education programme or as part of a continual professional development course, to undergo this learning. This chapter will also help you to recognise the drivers behind why many institutions are adding the NIPE education to their undergraduate education programmes for midwives. Roles in many areas of healthcare are changing; what were once deemed as extended roles are being viewed more and more as an expectation of newly qualified nurses and midwives. This move has been made to embrace the government ethos for the NHS, where midwives and nurses take on extended roles traditionally carried out by doctors (Department of Health, 2007, 2009).

The Nursing and Midwifery Council (NMC) are modernising the standards for the education and training of nurses and midwives, so that they will be equipped with the skills and knowledge they need to practise now, and in the future. As part of this ongoing discussion the consideration of what will be included in the new midwifery and nursing curricula due for publication in 2020 is important. Skills that are currently viewed as continued professional development, such as mentorship and nurse prescribing, are being considered as part of undergraduate education, as is the NIPE role. The reasons for these discussions and modifications have been linked to the healthcare landscape transformation; it has been decided that the nursing and midwifery standards need adjustment to keep up with the pace of change. If you are a student on an undergraduate education programme that incorporates the NIPE, you first need to, so this guide recognises that students may well be at varied points in their experience and learning. Yearley et al. (2017) found in their study that, of the 58 education institutions contacted in the UK, 40 (68.9%) completed the questionnaire, a quarter (25.0%) stated that NIPE training was at the time included in their pre-registration midwifery programmes, 37.5% reported plans to implement it within the next 2–5 years and 30.0% had no plans to do so (Yearley et al., 2017). It might be that other professionals with whom you are working clinically might have accessed this training as a further continuing professional development (CPD) professional qualification once working as a registered midwife or nurse.

Higher education institutions have been offering CPD courses related to the NIPE for over a decade now, and are well established. The professional carrying out the NIPE can be any practitioner who has received the relevant education and is deemed clinically competent. What was once deemed a role for paediatricians has now become the role of other professionals (Lumsden, 2005). At the time of publication, there is no recognised standard for this education, which includes the number of assessed clinical examinations necessary to be deemed proficient and competent. Currently this number is decided by individual higher education institutions, and again you might find diversity among your fellow practitioners if they completed their qualification at a different university. The number of academic credits awarded to the NIPE qualification can again vary because there is no national directive for this (Rogers et al., 2015).

Motivation for NIPE education

The professionals trained to complete the NIPE are usually midwives, one of the medical team or neonatal nurses. Although their training might differ in that nurses and midwives will attend a specific educational course related solely to the NIPE, the medical team have this training embedded within their medical education (Simms, 2005). From the author's observation, medical staff often learn skills from their midwifery and advanced neonatal nurse practitioner colleagues. Jones (2014) highlighted that some doctors may see the newborn examination as a task-oriented, physical screening tool, attributable to their traditional, medical model of healthcare, in which midwives and nurses have been noted as viewing this interaction not only as an opportunity for screening but also a chance to offer health promotion. Whoever carries out the examination, they must follow the same guidance in relation to what is examined and what referrals are being made. There has been an increase in the number of midwives and neonatal nurses carrying out the NIPE role in recent years for a number of reasons, one of which was the changes to the medical workforce working hours. Another reason was the recognition that, by supporting further development of teams, this can in fact have an effect on recruitment and retention. Workplace empowerment has been shown to be an important factor in creating a positive work environment for staff, therefore having a contributory impact on staff burnout and turnover (Nedd, 2006;

Laschinger et al., 2009). Laschinger et al. (1999, 2001, 2003, 2004, 2009) have produced many papers exploring empowerment in the workplace and how this can have positive effects on job satisfaction. It is evident from the research explored that the degree of control that staff perceive they have, related to the conditions of their work, is linked to the satisfaction that they feel. Nedd (2006) noted that, by creating a structure where nurses and midwives have access to opportunity, they can increase empowerment which in turn can improve efficiency of the workplace, thereby offering greater job satisfaction. Lumsden (2005) and Steele (2007) found that, by promoting the role of newborn examination, there can be an increase in job satisfaction which can aid midwifery retention (Jones, 2014). So, by supporting staff to develop, and embrace, new roles such as the NIPE this can ultimately have an impact on how empowered they feel. Studies by Bloomfield et al. (2003) and Hayes et al. (2003) propose that the examination of the newborn role for midwives sustains autonomy, as well as job satisfaction. The inclusion of the NIPE into many undergraduate programmes additionally evidences a shift in the challenges of financial support for CPD provision, which has been significantly reduced and is therefore less available (Jones, 2016). This has no doubt had an impact on the views on extended roles and the expectation of management teams within healthcare. Although acknowledging the critical contribution of CPD, it is essential that education of the NIPE is both cost-effective and fit for purpose (Rafferty et al., 2015). There is currently a drive to have some educational courses referred to as 'role essential qualifications'; because the push continues to increase the number of NIPE-qualified practitioners this may be a term that we will see used for NIPE education in the future. Rafferty et al. (2015) identified that, among nurses, barriers to CPD included workload pressures, difficulty in releasing staff and funding. It is likely that a similar situation exists in midwifery in relation to NIPE training (Rogers et al., 2015). The motivation for completing the NIPE education can be multifaceted, with the recognition that there is a distinct clinical need for more practitioners to be trained and available, to ensure both the efficiency of the national screening programme and the proficiency of discharge, in addition to supporting the development of new NIPE practitioners. However, the motivation for the practitioners themselves to complete the education programme can be linked to the intrinsic need to access further development and role improvement.

Midwives and the NIPE role

Historically, the NIPE has been predominantly performed by medical teams; however, in recent years the junior doctor role has been affected by changes in working time directives (European Commission, 2000). This has resulted in a reduction in junior doctors available to perform the NIPE, hence requiring midwives and nurses to embrace this role. Ultimately this has led to an increase in midwives and neonatal nurses accessing NIPE CPD modules (Jones and

Furber, 2017). It has long been argued that this was a natural progression and, in fact, the NIPE should very much be part of the midwifery role because it embodies the known benefits of continuity of carer as outlined in the NHS National Maternity Review (NHS England, 2016). There has been encouraging evidence that mothers have been positive about this role being carried out by midwives because the health promotion aspect of this examination has proved extremely beneficial (Bloomfield et al., 2003). The EMREN Study suggested that not only was mother's satisfaction improved when midwives performed the NIPE on postnatal wards, but also midwives undertaking this procedure could result in financial savings of up to £2.5 million nationally (Townsend et al., 2004). The Healthy Child Programme (Department of Health and Social Care, 2009), NIPE Programme (Department of Health, 2008), and now the 2018 Public Health England programme standards for the NIPE and National Institute for Health and Care Excellence (NICE, 2006) guidelines have all provided impetus for change to how the NIPE is now approached, not solely as a physical screen, but in the context of the assessment framework, providing the infant with the best chances in life, by placing increased importance on social and emotional welfare (Jones, 2014). The NIPE has long been seen as an 'added value' part of the midwife's role (Townsend et al., 2004). Historically, this was an enhanced role, meaning that midwives would undertake a period of post-registration theory and practical education to gain the qualification and skills; however, it is becoming more popular among undergraduate midwifery programmes. This, however, requires qualified NIPE mentors available to support the learning of both CPD and undergraduate learners. The age profile of the midwifery workforce is another compounding factor affecting the number of experienced NIPE-trained practitioners available and has added impetus for the NIPE education to be part of undergraduate midwifery education. Blake (2012) argued that incorporating the NIPE into undergraduate education is appropriate because there is no requirement for experience as it is education and assessment of competence that are the priority.

Research has identified that midwives performing the role offer benefits to women, the midwives themselves and the maternity service in which they work (Hutcherson, 2010). Indeed, in addition to increased continuity of care, job satisfaction and more efficient use of resources, examinations performed by midwives have been shown to be at least as effective as those of junior doctors. Midwives are in an ideal position to offer mothers and their families advice, in relation to both, making healthy choices for the best possible start for their infant, and to offer reassurance. In addition to the benefits when midwives perform this role, there has been an increase in neonatal teams, encouraging neonatal nurses to train to become NIPE practitioners, and it is firmly embedded in some workforce plans (Jones and Ashworth, 2016). Neonatal nurses are being increasingly viewed as another key team member in a prime position to carry out this role on postnatal wards.

There has been an array of documents and reports published, which direct the way in which teams working in the NHS function, and the inclusion of added skills within roles. The distinction between what parts of the NIPE should be the medical responsibility, and what parts the midwifery/nursing responsibility, is often blurred and can be driven by local guidance. One area, however, that has been clearly identified as being beneficial to both patients and professionals alike is the expansion of professional skills, with more nurses and midwives embracing enhanced roles (Jones and Ashworth, 2016).

Additional workforce pressures, such as the working time directive for junior doctors (European Commission, 2000), have provided the impetus for many maternity services increasingly seeking midwives who can carry out this role, thereby creating a normative culture that the NIPE should be part of midwifery care, rather than the previous medical model. This was first highlighted as an option in 2004 by Townsend et al. (2004) who suggested that midwives completing the NIPE would reduce overall health service costs and decrease the need for medical resources. Through the recognition of the change in service need, and on the basis of publications such as *Midwifery 2020* (2010), higher education institutions have begun to implement significant changes to midwifery education, including incorporation of the NIPE into the realm of pre-registration education. However, an important note is that increasing emphasis is being placed on the competence of all practitioners performing this area of practice, and that consistency for both education and competence assessment should a priority (Rogers et al., 2015). For students qualifying from midwifery education programmes with skills or theoretical education in relation to the NIPE, and for practitioners who may need to revisit the NIPE after a period of no practice, this guide will lead you through the step-by-step approach to the examination.

References

Blake, D. (2012). Newborn examination: the student's role? *British Journal of Midwifery*, **20**: 892–6.

Bloomfield, L., Townsend, J. and Rogers, C. (2003). A qualitative study exploring junior paediatricians', midwives', GPs' and mothers' experiences and views of the examination of the newborn infant. *Midwifery*, **19**(1): 37–45.

Department of Health (2007). *Maternity Matters: Choice, Access and Continuity of Care in a Safe Service*. London: The Stationery Office.

Department of Health (2008). *The Child Health Programme: Pregnancy and the First Five Years of Life*. London: Department for Children, Schools and Families.

Department of Health (2009). *Delivering High Quality Midwifery Care: The Priorities, pportunities and Challenges for Midwives*. London: The Stationery Office.

Department of Health and Social Care (2009). Healthy Child Programme: from 5 to 19 years old. Available at www.gov.uk/government/publications/healthy-child-programme-5-to-19-years-old (accessed 25 September 2018).

European Commission (2000). Directive 2000/34/EC of the European Parliament and of the Council of 22 June 2000. *Official Journal of the European Communities*, L195: 41–5.

Hayes, J., Dave, S., and Rogers, C. (2003). A national survey in England of the routine examination of the newborn. *Midwifery*, **19**: 277–84.

Hutcherson, A. (2010). Critical reflection on a midwife's development and practice in relation to examination of the newborn. *Midwives* December/January: 1–9.

Jones, L. (2014). Examination of the newborn – medical or holistic screening tool? *MIDIRS Midwifery Digest*, **24**(1): 93–8.

Jones, T. (2016). Changes to professional development, *British Journal of Midwifery*, **24**(6): 386.

Jones, T. and Ashworth, C. (2016). How the enhanced neonatal nurse practitioner role has been integral to one tertiary units workforce plan and service delivery. *Journal of Neonatal Nursing*, **22**: 147–51.

Jones, T. and Furber, C. (2017). Incorporating the theoretical aspects of the Newborn Infant Physical Examination into undergraduate midwifery education: The University of Manchester experience. *British Journal of Midwifery*, **25**(9): doi. org/10.12968/bjom.2017.25.9.593.

Laschinger, H.K.S., Wong, C., McMahon, L. and Kaufmann, C. (1999). Leader behaviour impact on staff nurse empowerment, job tension, and work effectiveness. *Journal of Nursing Administration*, **29**(5): 28–39.

Laschinger, H.K.S., Finegan, J. and Shamian, J. (2001). The impact of workplace empowerment, organizational trust on staff nurses' work satisfaction and organizational commitment. *Health Care Management Review*, **26**(3): 7–23.

Laschinger, H.K.S., Almost, J. and Tuer-Hodes, D. (2003). Workplace empowerment and magnet hospital characteristics: Making the link. *Journal of Nursing Administration*, **33**: 410–22.

Laschinger, H.K.S., Finegan, J.E., Shamian, J. and Wilk, P. (2004). A longitudinal analysis of the impact of workplace empowerment on work satisfaction. *Journal of Organizational Behavior*, **25**: 527–45.

Laschinger, H.K.S., Leiter, M., Day, A. and Gilin, D. (2009). Workplace empowerment, incivility, and burnout: Impact on staff nurse recruitment and retention outcomes. *Journal of Nursing Management*, **17**: 302–11.

Lumsden, H. (2005). Midwives' experience of examination of the newborn as an additional aspect of their role: A qualitative study. *MIDIRS Midwifery Digest*, **15**: 450–7.

Midwifery 2020 (2010). Midwifery 2020 programme: delivering expectations. Available at: www.gov.uk/government/publications/midwifery-2020-delivering-expectations (accessed 17 January 2018).

National Institute for Health and Care Excellence (2006). *Routine Postnatal Care of Women and Their Babies. NICE Clinical Guideline 37*. Available at: www.nice.org.uk/guidance/CG37 (accessed 25 April 2019).

Nedd, N. (2006). Perceptions of empowerment and intent to stay. *Nursing Economics*, **24**(1): 13.

NHS England (2016). *National Maternity Review. National Maternity Review: Better Births: Improving outcomes of maternity services in England – A five year forward view for maternity care*. London: NHS England.

Public Health England (2018). NHS Newborn Physical and Infant Examination Programme (NIPE). NIPE Programme Standards. Available at: www.gov.uk/government/publications/newborn-and-infant-physical-examination-screening-standards (accessed May 2018).

Rafferty, A.M., Xyrichis, A. and Caldwell, C. (2015). Post-graduate education and career pathways in nursing: A policy brief. Report to Lord Willis, Independent Chair of the Shape of Caring Review. National Nursing Research Unit, King's College, London.

Rogers, C., Yearley, C. and Beeton, K. (2015). National survey of current practice standards for the newborn and infant physical examination. *British Journal of Midwifery*, **23**: 862–73.

Simms, M. (2005). Midwives and the neonatal examination. *British Journal of Midwifery*, **8**(5): 21–3.

Steele, D. (2007). Examining the newborn: Why don't midwives use their skills. *Midwifery*, **15**: 748–52.

Townsend, J., Wolke, D. and Hayes, J. (2004). Routine examination of the newborn: The EMREN study. Evaluation of an extension of the midwife role including a randomised control trial of appropriately trained midwives and paediatric house officers. *Health Technology Assessment*, **8**(14): 1–73.

Yearley, C., Rogers, C. and Jay, A. (2017). Including the Newborn Physical Examination (NIPE) in the pre-registration midwifery curriculum: National survey. *British Journal of Midwifery*, **25**(1): 26–32.

3 Communication skills in healthcare

Tracey Jones

Introduction

Clinical practice commands the application of knowledge, skills and values in diverse combinations. For a newborn infant physical examination (NIPE) practitioner, communication is a key facet of the skills that assure that the NIPE is being effectively completed; it can encompass communication with the infant, the parents and the wider multidisciplinary team, as well as recording the examination. This chapter considers communication in the context of 'patient-centred care', care focused on the need of the individual. With regard to the care of the newborn/infant, the related concepts of 'family-centred care' (POPPY Steering Group 2009) and 'family integrated care' (Patel et al., 2018) are important, emphasising the extent to which elements of communication in the NIPE will be directed towards the parents.

Although the NIPE may present challenges to the resourcefulness of the practitioner, it is an excellent opportunity, in a protected timescale and environment, to observe, assess and address complex needs, such as public health, safeguarding, emotional attachment, and the social and emotional welfare of the parents, and to attain the best outcomes in life for the child, reaffirming that the midwife and neonatal nurse are ideally placed to carry out this role (Jones, 2014). It is recognised that the arena of midwifery care is challenged both in the ratio of patients to midwives and the speed-to-patient turnover. The lack of time available when caring for women in normal midwifery postnatal care can mean that women may be left with unanswered questions related to ongoing care; having your attention during the NIPE is often an ideal opportunity to ask them.

About this chapter

After studying this chapter you should be able to:

- recognise relevant benchmarks and standards for effective communication
- identify potential barriers to effective communication in the NIPE
- use models of effective communication to guide your practice during the NIPE

Definitions: communication and effective communication

The Department of Health (currently the Department of Health and Social Care) document *Essence of Care 2010* (Department of Health, 2010, p. 7), in its benchmarks for communication, defines 'communication' as:

> a process that involves a meaningful exchange between at least two people to convey facts, needs, opinions, thoughts, feelings or other information through both verbal and non-verbal means, including face-to-face exchanges and the written word.

Essence of Care 2010 sets benchmarks for 'effective communication' as an agreed, person-centred outcome for 'people' (people requiring care) and carers. These benchmarks include:

- *Interpersonal skills*, to be demonstrated by all staff
- *Opportunity for communication*, which requires an acceptable time and environment
- *Assessment of communication needs*, which should be regular and may trigger the provision of additional support
- *Information sharing*, which requires accessible and accurate information to be actively shared with people and carers
- *Empowerment for people and carers to communicate their needs*: staff must make it possible for people and carers to express their needs at any time
- *Valuing people's and carers' expertise and contribution*: staff must value, record and act on these.

Relevant NMC standards: communication and referral

The Nursing and Midwifery Council (NMC, 2015) Code sets the standards that registered nurses and midwives must uphold. Sections 7 and 8 are detailed as part of the standard for practising effectively:

Section 7, *'Communicating clearly'*, requires nurses and midwives to do the following:

7.1 use terms that people in your care, colleagues and the public can understand

7.2 take reasonable steps to meet people's language and communication needs, providing, wherever possible, assistance to those who need help to communicate their own or other people's needs

7.3 use a range of verbal and non-verbal communication methods, and consider cultural sensitivities, to better understand and respond to people's personal and health needs

7.4   check people's understanding from time to time to keep misunder-standing or mistakes to a minimum, and

7.5   be able to communicate clearly and effectively in English.

Section 8 of the Code, 'Work cooperatively', includes the requirements that nurses and midwives must:

8.1   respect the skills, expertise and contributions of your colleagues, refer-ring matters to them when appropriate

8.2   maintain effective communication with colleagues.

Communication in the NIPE

Successful communication in the NIPE requires the practitioner to attend to the parents' needs for information and emotional care, while completing and recording a complex and through examination of the child that is enhanced by the information obtained from the parents.

We discuss appropriate models and principles of communication that will empower you to meet the relevant NMC standards and Department of Health benchmarks, and identify and overcome barriers to effective communication.

Models of communication

Models of communication can be used in healthcare to interpret behaviour and to indicate good practice. Over the past 70 years they have evolved from *linear* to *interactive* and *transactional* models.

Linear models, such as that of Shannon and Weaver (1949), are based on the concept of a [human] 'sender' 'encoding' and then 'transmitting' a 'message' to a [human] 'receiver' who 'decodes' the message, with, in the Shannon and Weaver model, 'noise', such as audio stimuli, interfering with the effectiveness of the transmission. Observations of noisy ward environments can suggest a straightforward application of this model to healthcare settings. However, linear models are seen as failing to consider the social, cultural and other environmental contexts of communication and as ignoring the impact of com-munication on the 'receiver'.

Interactive models, for example that of Schramm (1955), regard communica-tion as a process of *social interaction*. Schramm's model identifies the importance of the *fields of experience* of the sender and receiver of the message. This describes the language and other experiences that allow the participants in social inter-action to encode and decode messages. An example application to healthcare would identify the problems experienced when professionals in consultation use jargon and other language outside the experience of patients and carers.

Transactional models of communication, for example that described by Wood (2009), add the dimension of recognising that communicators may *simultaneously* send and receive messages: a 'speaker' will typically be scanning their audience for feedback to see how their message is being received, thus also acting as a 'receiver'. Transactional models also take into account the *dynamic* nature of communication, recognising that modes of communication between individuals change over time as the relationship between those individuals develops, for example with the development of trust in a nurse–patient relationship. Furthermore, these models also consider more widely the 'systems', or 'contexts', within which communication takes place. These contexts include personal and shared experiences, cultural influences and formal contexts such as hospital settings and health procedures, and again there is an awareness of the dynamic nature of communication; contexts can change over time. The concept of 'noise' in transactional models encompasses all forms of interference with the communication, including such cognitive processes in the communicators as prejudice.

In the context of the NIPE examination, an awareness of the transactional model of communication is the most useful. For example, as a health professional giving information you should actively look for feedback from patients to understand how well your message is being understood; we consider this in more detail in the section on active listening. The *contexts* of the examination may include the parents' recent and past experiences (negative or positive) in contact with health services, and their concerns about the wellbeing of their child. These must be borne in mind if the practitioner is to provide appropriate informative and supportive care. If you are caring for a family who have previously lost an infant, you might have to make additional considerations, perhaps making a little more time available, or it might be that you need to involve the medical team or neonatal outreach should the family warrant the loan of an apnoea alarm. The parents will be understandably concerned and anxious, so the way in which you communicate will relieve their concerns. Mills et al. (2014) found, in their metasynthesis aimed at improving understanding of parents' experiences of maternity care in pregnancy after stillbirth or neonatal death, that the death of a previous infant significantly affected parents' experiences. They described how their subsequent pregnancies were characterised by heightened anxiety and fear, and suggest that individual experiences are shaped by a multiplicity of internal and external factors; emotions are often intensified or reawakened in subsequent pregnancies. As a NIPE practitioner, having knowledge of parents' previous experiences will equip you in preparation for any questions or concerns that might arise. The importance of examining the maternal notes before embarking on the NIPE is covered in depth in Chapter 6.

Effective communication in healthcare practice

A considerable body of evidence suggests both the importance of effective communication in healthcare and the extent to which healthcare professionals (HCPs) have failed to meet the communication needs of patients and carers.

The literature review by Charlton et al. (2008) identifies the difference between *biomedical* and *biopsychosocial* modes of communication by HCPs. Biomedical (traditional medical) communication is described as being essential directive, with little regard being given to patient input. Biopsychosocial, or patient-centred, communication is described as having a basis of partnership with the patient and carers, and features more open-ended discussion.

Biomedical communication is identified in Charlton et al.'s (2008) review with negative patient outcomes. These include:

- patients and families suing the HCP, which was more likely to happen if the patient felt ignored or rushed by the HCP
- poor treatment adherence, caused by poor understanding of instructions
- low levels of patient satisfaction leading to poor patient-to-HCP communication
- low levels of patient self-care.

Conversely, biopsychosocial communication is associated in the same review with positive patient outcomes. These include:

- high levels of treatment adherence
- improved pain control
- improved symptom resolution
- increased patient satisfaction.

Analysing papers that evaluate the communication styles of nurse practitioners, Charlton et al. (2008) conclude that biopsychosocial/patient-centred modes of communication are associated with improved patient satisfaction, improved treatment adherence and improved patient health.

McCabe and Timmins (2006) identify attentive listening and information giving, with a patient-centred focus, as key communication skills for a biopsychosocial approach. We shall consider how you can best employ these skills for effective communication in the NIPE.

Giving information

Information demands of the NIPE

Information about the NIPE should be provided to parents antenatally and before the infant examination, and parents must be informed of the findings of each examination (Public Health England, 2018). Before commencing the examination you will be required to clarify with the parents any abnormalities found in the maternal case notes. This not only demonstrates that you have started with a thorough background, but also assures the parents that you are competent and knowledgeable. You might need to question any areas that were not clear or may well have been missed. It is important to have this discussion before disturbing the infant because it is more beneficial to extract further information when the parents are fully focused and not distracted by their unsettled infant. You will be able to gather a large amount of information from the mother about feeding volumes and tolerances: what has the output been like, and is she concerned about anything?

You may choose to discuss the findings of the examination with the parents as you proceed, and will certainly need to summarise these at the end of the examination. (Some practitioners prefer to verbalise each part of the examination, explaining what they are examining as they proceed. For example, they might explain about the red reflex in the eye, and why this is often a challenging part of the examination to achieve but is vital to completion. As the parents' support may be needed with this part of the examination, it is useful for them to understand the importance of persisting until both eyes have been examined successfully. The practitioner may also explain why they are performing the cardiovascular examination at the start of the NIPE, while the infant is settled and asleep, rather than performing the examination in the systematic way. Informing the parents of the potential distress the infant might well vocalise when the practitioner examines the hips not only prepares them, and reduces their concern, but may also give you more confidence, in that they are supportive of your examination and assist to settle the infant.)

If a referral is indicated, you will need to provide parents with an explanation of the detected abnormality, the reason for the referral and an indication of how the referral will progress.

You will need to ensure as far as possible that the parents have sufficiently understood the information that you have given to them.

Caress (2003) outlines some of the factors that may impair or facilitate health information giving. With regard to the recipients of the information, she points out that:

- information may not be understood because the recipients find it too complex or hard to read
- information may not be understood because the recipients are too anxious to process it
- the recipients of the information may choose to disbelieve it, either because the information (or the person delivering it) does not seem credible, or because the information does not fit in with their beliefs.

The individual's ability to understand health information can be equated to their degree of 'health literacy'. The World Health Organization (Dodson et al., 2015) define this as:

> ...the personal characteristics and social resources needed for individuals and communities to access, understand, appraise and use information and services to make decisions about health. Health literacy includes the capacity to communicate, assert and enact these decisions.

Low levels of health literacy are found in a surprisingly large percentage of the population; Rowlands et al. (2015) found that 41% of English adults (18–65) do not have sufficient health literacy, and 61% do not have sufficient health *numeracy*, to understand health information. Clearly, therefore, HCPs need to ensure that their information is directed at an appropriate level of complexity for most people to understand (Health Education England, n.d.). The Pfizer health literacy website for health professionals (Pfizer, n.d.) suggests that information should be presented in plain language and in manageable amounts:

- Assess the current level of knowledge in the person before presenting information, so that you can present the information at the appropriate level of complexity
- Medical jargon should be avoided
- Statements should be as specific as possible
- Avoid terms (e.g. 'stool') that have different meanings in healthcare and everyday settings
- Present information in the form of key points
- Provide additional information to take away in written or other formats.

Caress (2003) identifies other groups who may find health information difficult to process. The diverse, multicultural nature of the UK means that we cannot presume that the preferred language of the parents present during the NIPE will be spoken English. Therefore, it may be necessary to involve an interpreter throughout the examination, translating to another spoken or signed language. Parents may also require specialist support for their sensory impairments or learning disabilities. There are varied systems and policies in place to support these services, and you should explore and become familiar with these in your area of practice, ensuring that you can arrange appropriate support in advance of the NIPE.

The use of a professional interpreter is important to ensure that translation is carried out accurately and impartially. Your practice area will have its own policies in place for interpretation, but these will typically caution against the use of the following in NIPEs:

- Family members, who may interpret inaccurately because they are untrained; they may distort or filter communication due to embarrassment and personal or cultural sensitivities
- Children, who lack the linguistic and cognitive development to act as interpreters in sensitive and stressful situations
- Colleagues, whose use of time to interpret may be considered inappropriate and who are not typically trained in interpretation.

Active listening

Fischer-Lokou et al. (2016) propose that listening is essential if communication is to be effective. They suggest that the skills of 'active listening' in HCPs improve patient care and satisfaction. The suite of skills referred to as 'active listening' derive from Carl Rogers' (1951) humanist psychology, and have been deployed in a range of disciplines. Weger et al. (2010) identify three common elements:

1 The active listener communicates that they are providing unconditional attention to the speaker
2 The active listener restates (without making judgements) what they feel to be the content and the feelings in the speaker's message, and by paraphrasing demonstrates that they understand the intended message
3 The active listener asks questions to encourage the speaker to expand; Zofi and Meltzer (2007) emphasise that active listening encourages two-way communication.

For the NIPE examiner, the use of active listening allows you to check the parents' level of understanding of your message, identify unspoken anxieties and provide the parents with the opportunity to voice concerns. It is essential that you recognise that, for example, parents are not participating in the examination or that they are significantly quiet; the time allocated to the NIPE is a superlative opportunity to address any concerns that the parents may well have or just to offer some professional support. You might well find that the discussion moves away from the NIPE to other topic areas that the parents have wanted to discuss but have not had the opportunity to broach with other members of the team.

Robertson (2005) sees active listening as attending to the complete verbal and non-verbal message that the person is conveying. She suggests that this can be demonstrated by, among other technique, the following.

Attentive body language

- Posture that shows engagement, by being oriented towards the speaker
- Appropriate facial expressions, which indicate interest and engagement rather than boredom, distaste, alarm or a need to be elsewhere
- Appropriate eye contact, which indicates interest and engagement but does not threaten by staring.

Following skills

- Minimal verbal 'encouragers', such as 'Mmm', or 'I see', that encourage open communication
- Attentive silences that encourage open communication by demonstrating that you are listening and are giving space for the other person to speak.

Reflecting skills

- Paraphrasing: putting what the other person has said in new words to demonstrate that you are listening and have understood
- Reflecting back feelings and content.

Similarly, Egan (1990) uses the acronym 'SOLER' to describe a set of behaviours that help to demonstrate attention:

- Sitting attentively (at an angle towards the person with whom you are conversing)
- Open posture (not defensively crossing your arms)
- Leaning forward (to express interest, and the better to pick up non-verbal clues and quiet verbal communication)
- Eye contact (to express interest, avoiding staring)
- Relaxed body language (to demonstrate that you are not in too much of a hurry to hear what the other person has to say).

To promote active listening, the Pfizer (n.d.) health literacy website encourages the health professional to:

- use open-ended questions, such as 'What questions do you want to ask me?', rather than closed questions such as 'Have you got any questions for me?', which are more likely to lead to a negative response
- use the 'teach back' technique to ask the patient/carer to demonstrate that they have understood by repeating their understanding of the information.

In the potentially emotionally fraught context of childbirth, it is important to remember to control your own non-verbal communication during the NIPE. Puzzled or concerned expressions on your part may be picked up and amplified by already concerned parents and exacerbate their anxieties, as well as potentially communicating doubts about your ability to manage the situation. Working with your mentor will enable you to develop communication skills specifically dealing with situations where an abnormality has been found. The sensitive nature by which any concern or referral is communicated can not only have immediate effects but also instil long-term memories for parents. Nuzum et al. (2014) noted that the way in which professionals communicate bad news to parents is remembered in painstaking detail, often revisited as parents seek to understand their loss. They clearly documented that the sensitivity of how news is broken to parents is often recalled as part of the overall memory of experience. Parents appreciate when clinicians offer time when breaking bad news. In addition to these findings the clarity of words used is also of equal importance; it is vital that parents understand plainly what is being said to them. The use of medical terms can often be confusing and mystifying to parents, sometimes making the information sound more serious than it actually is. It is well documented that the way in which information is imparted impacts on the experiences of parents and that good communication when bad news is being given is of the utmost importance (Fallowfield and Jenkins, 2004; Kelley and Trinidad, 2012). Finding an abnormality during the NIPE will be covered in more depth throughout the book.

Using a combination of these active listening techniques will allow you to gain as much useful information from the parents as possible, while allowing them to voice their own concerns freely.

Communication in the NIPE: barriers and solutions

Tables 3.1 and 3.2 use the models of communication and theories of effective communication to:

1   identify possible barriers to effective communication in the NIPE
2   identify pathways to effective communication in the NIPE.

Table 3.1 Possible barriers to effective communication in the newborn infant physical examination (NIPE)	
Environmental 'noise'	The setting for the NIPE does not exclude sounds or visual distractions
Parents' language 'context'	The parents have a low level of health literacy/numeracy, and/or do not have a native command of English and/or have a degree of learning disability
Parents' emotional 'context'	The parents' levels of anxiety about their child's health and/or the hospital setting make it difficult for them to process information and/or ask appropriate questions
Parents' sensory 'context'	The parents have sensory impairments or are deaf and/or blind; the healthcare professional fails to make adjustments to accommodate this
Healthcare professional fails to orient parents	The healthcare professional fails to provide a rationale and description of the NIPE procedure at the beginning of the examination, making the process harder to understand and potentially increasing parents' anxiety levels
Poor 'encoding' of information by healthcare professional	The healthcare professional message is incoherent and/or uses medical language beyond the health literacy of the parents
Healthcare professional displays poor 'active listening' skills	The healthcare professional fails to use active listening to • check the parents' understanding • establish any parental concerns • encourage questions from the parents • indicate to the parents that she understands their needs

Table 3.2 Effective communication during the newborn infant physical examination (NIPE)

Secure adequate time for the NIPE. If necessary, make reasonable adjustments to extend the time for the examination, for example if the parents require an interpreter

Use an appropriate physical environment for the NIPE. The examination should be taking place in a time-protected and private environment

If necessary, ensure that a qualified interpreter is in place for the NIPE

Before commencing the NIPE, establish the parents' current understanding of the infant's wellbeing and allow discussion of any concerns. Gauge the parents' health literacy

Before commencing the NIPE, inform the parents of the purpose of the examination and how it will be carried out. Use active listening techniques to ensure that they have understood what is going to happen before obtaining their consent to the procedure

During the NIPE, if you choose to discuss the findings of the examination as you proceed, ensure that you use language appropriate to the health literacy of the parents and present the information in manageable amounts, point by point. Use active listening techniques to assess whether the parents understand your information and to pick up on unspoken concerns or anxiety on their part. Ensure that you maintain positive or neutral non-verbal communication, such as your facial expressions, in order not to alarm the parents

After completion of the NIPE, discuss the findings of the NIPE with the parents. Ensure that you use language appropriate to the health literacy of the parents and present the information in manageable amounts, point by point. Use active listening to ensure that they have understood the findings. Ensure that you encourage and respond to questions, using active listening techniques, even for what you may regard as a routine and normal examination

If the NIPE indicates that a referral is required, clearly explain to the parents the nature of the detected abnormality, the reason for the referral and how long the referral process may take. Ensure that you use language appropriate to the health literacy of the parents and present the information in manageable amounts, point by point. Use active listening techniques to ensure that they have understood this

References

Caress, A.-L. (2003). Giving information to patients. *Nursing Standard*, **17**(43): 47–54.

Charlton, C.R., Dearing, K.S., Berry, J.A. and Johnson, M.J. (2008). Nurse practitioners' communication styles and their impact on patient outcomes: An integrated literature review. *Journal of the American Academy of Nurse Practitioners*, **20**: 382–8.

Department of Health (2010). Essence of Care 2010. Benchmarks for the fundamental aspects of care. Available at https://assets.publishing.service.gov.uk/

government/uploads/system/uploads/attachment_data/file/216691/dh_119978. pdf (accessed 7 October 2018).

Dodson, S., Good, S. and Osborne, R.H. (2015). *Health Literacy Toolkit for Low- and Middle-income Countries: A series of information sheets to empower communities and strengthen health systems.* New Delhi: World Health Organization.

Egan, G. (1990). *The Skilled Helper: A systematic approach to effective helping,* 4th edn. Belmont, CA: Thomson Brooks/Cole Publishing Co.

Fallowfield, L. and Jenkins, V. (2004). Communicating sad, bad, and difficult news in medicine. *The Lancet,* **363**: 312–19.

Fischer-Lokou, J., Lamy, L., Guéguen, N. and Dubarry, A. (2016). Effects of active listening, reformulation, and imitation on mediator success: Preliminary results. *Psychological Reports,* **118**: 994–1010.

Health Education England (n.d.) Health literacy 'how to' guide. Available at: https:// healtheducationengland.sharepoint.com/:f:/g/Comms/Digital/EqkgGjdcNhdIuEs-FcobL3wBr7tLzYQnfg790Q1blIiyCA?e=FJzkD4 (accessed 7 October 2018).

Jones, L. (2014). Examination of the newborn – medical or holistic screening tool? *MIDIRS Midwifery Digest,* **24**(1): 93–8.

Kelley, M.C. and Trinidad, S.B. (2012). Silent loss and the clinical encounter: Parents' and physicians' experiences of stillbirth-a qualitative analysis. *BMC Pregnancy & Childbirth,* **12**: 137–51.

McCabe, C. and Timmins, F. (2006). *Communication Skills for Nursing Practice.* Basingstoke: Palgrave Macmillan.

Mills, T., Ricklesford, C., Cooke, A., Heazell, A.E.P., Whitworth, M. and Lavender, T. (2014). Parents' experiences and expectations of care in pregnancy after stillbirth or neonatal death: A metasynthesis. *British Journal of Obstetrics and Gynaecology,* **121**: 943–50.

Nursing and Midwifery Council (2015). *The Code. Professional Standards of Practice and Behaviour for Nurses and Midwives.* London: NMC.

Nuzum, D., Meaney, S. and O'Donoghue, K. (2014). Breaking bad news: The impact on parents. *Archives of Diseases in Childhood Fetal Neonatal,* **99**(Suppl 1): A1–180.

Patel, N., Ballantyne, A., Bowker, G., Weightman, J. and Weightman, S. (2018). Family integrated care: Changing the culture in the neonatal unit. *Archives of Diseases in Childhood,* **103**: 415–19.

Pfizer (n.d.). Health literacy (website). Available at: www.pfizer.com/health/literacy/ healthcare-professionals (accessed 7 October 2018).

POPPY Steering Group (2009). *Family-centred Care in Neonatal Units. A summary of research results and recommendations from the POPPY project.* London: NCT.

Public Health England (2018). Newborn and infant physical examination screening programme handbook. Available at: www.gov.uk/government/publications/ newborn-and-infant-physical-examination-programme-handbook/newborn-and-infant-physical-examination-screening-programme-handbook (accessed 7 October 2018).

Robertson, K. (2005). Active listening: More than just paying attention. *Australian Family Physician,* **34**: 1053–5.

Rogers, C.R. (1951). *Client-centered Therapy.* Boston, MA: Houghton-Mifflin.

Rowlands, G., Protheroe, J., Winkley, J., Richardson, M., Seed, P.T. and Rudd, R. (2015). A mismatch between population health literacy and the complexity of health information: an observational study. *British Journal of General Practice,* **65**: e379–86.

Shannon, C. and Weaver, W. (1949). *The Mathematical Theory of Communication.* Urbana, IL: University of Illinois Press.

Schramm, W. (1955). *The Process and Effects of Mass Communication.* Urbana, IL: University of Illinois Press.

Weger, H., Castle, G.R. and Emmett, M.C. (2010). Active listening in peer interviews: The influence of message paraphrasing on perceptions of listening skill. *International Journal of Listening*, **24**(1): 34–49.

Wood, J.T. (2009). *Communication in Our Lives*, 4th edn. Belmont, CA: Thomson-Wadsworth.

Zofi, Y. and Meltzer, S. (2007). Listening takes practice. *Nursing Homes Magazine*, May: 70–1.

Maternal factors that influence fetal development

Carol Mashhadi

Introduction

The relationship between mother and fetus is one of dependency because the fetus cannot survive without the mother in the early gestational weeks of pregnancy. Indeed, not only does it rely on the mother for nutrients and protection but also is directly influenced by any maternal factors that may ultimately determine the outcome of the pregnancy. With this in mind, this chapter explores the maternal factors that influence fetal development, taking into consideration obstetric, medical, social and environmental factors.

Most neonatal examinations performed will reveal nothing abnormal; however, a relatively small proportion will reveal elements of dysmorphia, many of which will be minor. The reasons for this, and degree of abnormality, are influenced by the event and stage of fetal development (Sadler, 2015). As a must be given to any maternal influences that may impact fetal/newborn outcomes. Family trends and traits also need to be considered, but not to the exclusion of variations that fall outside this influence.

The importance of good history taking (Public Health England, 2018), together with a comprehensive examination, cannot be emphasised enough because it raises NIPE practitioners' knowledge and vigilance during the assessment.

Figure 4.1 shows the stages of fetal development, potential outcomes and degree of morphology depending on the type of external factor.

Consideration is now given to individual elements, throughout the child-bearing continuum, that may influence fetal/newborn development. These are considered under the subheadings of early pregnancy/antepartum, intrapartum and postnatal period.

Early pregnancy/antepartum

Pregnancy extends from conception to birth, which means that there are significant potential opportunities for factors to impact fetal development.

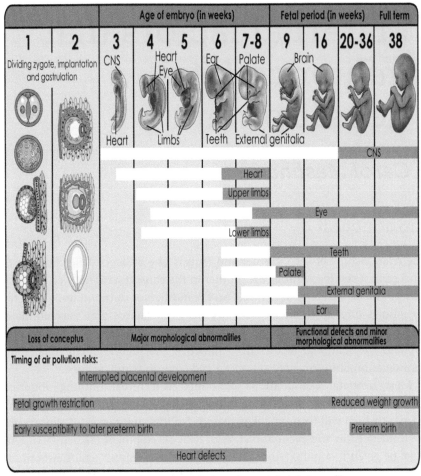

(Note: light grey bars indicate time periods when major morphological abnormalities can occur, while the dark grey bars correspond to periods at risk for minor abnormalities and functional defects

Figure 4.1
Embrology development

The most serious complications occur in the early embryonic phase between 3 and 8 weeks. Insults occurring within 2 weeks of fertilisation will have one of two outcomes: either survival or loss of the pregnancy (as highlighted in Figure 4.1). The reason for this is related to the development of the zygote, a fragile cell mass, which goes through significant changes during early development (Sadler, 2015). Any insult at this crucial stage of development will result in cell damage. If only a few cells are affected this may result in a minor or major anomaly dependent on what cells are affected (Sadler, 2015). It is rare to see anomalies in the final 9 weeks of development because this is recognised as a growth phase (see Figure 4.1).

CLINICAL TIP

Good history taking before the clinical assessment will offer you an understanding of the birth transition and highlight key areas for concern.

There is recognition that the demographics of the maternal population has changed significantly in recent years and more women with significantly complex needs are being supported through maternity services (National Institute for Health and Care Excellence (NICE, 2010), the consequence of this being the potential impact of their conditions on fetal development. Medical conditions such as diabetes and epilepsy all require a joint approach to care during pregnancy (NICE, 2010), in an attempt to safeguard the health and wellbeing of both the mother and the fetus.

Review of antenatal screening before the NIPE assessment will provide the practitioner with information to aid risk assessment of the fetus/newborn, and establish the appropriateness for midwife examination (Public Health England, 2018). Due to the potential for placental transmission of blood-borne viruses and maternal antibodies, NIPE practitioners need to check carefully any maternal serology during the antenatal period. The significance of blood group and rhesus factor, in relation to incompatibilities and neonatal haemolytic disease, is well recognised (Daniels and Bromilow, 2014). Early recognition and management are essential to prevent or reduce the effects of this condition.

THINK POINT

Consider how contracting a virus in pregnancy might affect the unborn fetus?

Blood-borne viruses, for example, human immunodeficiency virus (HIV) and hepatitis B, can be transferred to the fetus *in utero*; antiretroviral drugs for HIV should be offered to treat the mother. Keeping the viral load low will potentially reduce transmission (Royal College of Obstetrics and Gynaecologists [RCOG], 2010); in addition, newborn vaccination would be offered for hepatitis B in the postnatal period (NICE, 2014). Additional screening may also be offered for chlamydia infection, toxoplasmosis, varicella (chickenpox) and rubella, if the woman has had exposure during pregnancy. Fetal exposure and outcome are directly linked to the timing of the exposure. The earlier the exposure the greater the impact, which can range from spontaneous pregnancy loss, fetal brain and eye damage to varicella infection of the newborn (RCOG, 2015).

In the UK pre-pregnancy diabetes is one of the most common medical conditions influencing pregnancy; its prevalence has increased significantly in the last 20 years from 1.56 per 1000 pregnancies to 4.09 per 1000 pregnancies (Coton et al., 2016). The condition has associations with complications in pregnancy and adverse outcomes for the fetus, with an affiliated increase in spontaneous abortion, congenital anomalies and perinatal mortality (MBRRACE-UK) (Department of Health, 2017). During early pregnancy and antenatal periods, the aim is to maintain maternal blood glucose levels within the range recommended for all individuals with type 1 diabetes, to reduce adverse outcomes (NICE, 2015a). Joint antenatal appointments with specialist input should be provided alongside the routine care for pregnancy (NICE, 2010, 2015b). Recommendations for a change of medication will also be advised when the likely benefits for improved blood glucose control outweigh the potential for harm to the developing fetus (NICE, 2015a); for NIPE practitioners, vigilant appraisal of documentation is essential to ascertain any risk related to this condition.

Ongoing antenatal screening should include an individualised approach to care, which may incorporate ultrasound scans to detect structural anomalies, fetal growth and amniotic fluid volume, alongside Doppler recording and fetal heart monitoring (NICE, 2015a), all of which can be reviewed by the practitioner before the NIPE assessment.

CLINICAL TIP

Have you made a thorough check of the clinical notes for preconceptual advice? Do you need to ask the woman about preconceptual care?

Similarly, women with epilepsy planning their pregnancy should seek preconception care because it is recognised that the risk of congenital malformations in the fetus is low if they are not exposed to antiepileptic drugs (AEDs) in this period. However, when this is not possible women need to be informed that potential fetal congenital abnormalities may be influenced by the type, number and dose of AEDs, particularly the long-term impact on neurological development in the newborn (RCOG, 2016).

THINK POINT

Examine your clinical guidance on what types of AEDs are being recommended in pregnancy?

Joint management between clinicians specialising in this condition and obstetricians is advised, to optimise the best outcomes for both the mother and the fetus. The benefits of shared decision-making around choice and dose of AEDs to control seizures, balanced against the risk to the fetus, are crucial (RCOG, 2016).

As outlined there is clear evidence of the effect of direct maternal transmission of infections or impact of maternal medical conditions on fetal development. However, social and environmental factors also play a key role in influencing fetal outcomes in early development.

From more commonly observed smoking to the misuse of alcohol, prescribed and non-prescribed substances all have the potential to cause anomalies in the fetus, depending on the timing, frequency, dose and type of substance used (see Figure 4.1). NICE (2010) recommendations for care of women with complex needs highlighted the requirement for access to multi-agency care, partnership working and clear referral pathways, a factor closely associated with the NIPE (Public Health England, 2016). The need for women to be treated with kindness, respect and dignity is paramount, and above all else clear communication and informed decision-making should be central to the NIPE practitioner.

There are many similarities with the effects of different substances on pregnancy and fetal development, from reduced fertility and miscarriage through to preterm birth, growth restriction and stillbirth. Alcohol can be acutely problematic with fetal alcohol syndrome (FAS) or fetal alcohol spectrum disorder (Sadler, 2015) potentially causing long-term effects. Neurological defects and mental capacity, congenital abnormalities and physical facial anomalies have been recognised as an effect of drinking during pregnancy and associated with FAS (Department of Health, 2016). For the NIPE practitioner, recognition and knowledge of normal neurological behaviour and facial structure will support the assessment and potential detection of anomalies.

Prescribed and non-prescribed substances, for example cocaine, benzodiazepines and opiates, are also associated with defects in neurological development, congenital abnormalities of the heart, limbs, genitourinary system and cleft palate (Behnke and Smith, 2013; Sadler, 2015; Cleft Lip and Palate Association, n.d.). Although some of these abnormalities may be externally visible and, therefore, not assessed by midwives, some may be detected during the NIPE assessment, particularly in relation to heart anomalies (Public Health England, 2016). This reinforces the need for effective history taking and documentation review before assessment.

Although the above elements can be avoided, women may be unaware of environmental factors that may also have significant impacts on pregnancy and fetal development. The use of pesticides, radioactivity, heavy metals and even anaesthetic gases can be invisible to the general population and may have little or no effect or long-term outcomes; however, for the developing pregnancy and fetus the effects can be linked to miscarriage and congenital abnormality (Sadler, 2015).

THINK POINT

What dietary advice and precautions are given to women pre-conceptually and during pregnancy?

As previously stated the demographics of women are changing. With the increase in migration, asylum seeking or refugee status, there is a group of women who may have difficulty reading or speaking the local language. The limitation in language may reduce the chances of these woman accessing appropriate care and advice, potentially putting themselves and their fetus at risk of complication (NICE, 2010). Although NIPE practitioners may see these women only after childbirth, it is vital that communication is supported by interpreters, if necessary when reviewing clinical notes, should there be a need for further questions (NICE, 2010).

THINK POINT

What is your current local trust guidance on use of interpreters?

Intrapartum

As previously outlined many of the fetal/newborn developmental impacts will be closely associated with the early pregnancy/antenatal period due to the close maternal links. However, the intrapartum period can have significant long-term effects on the fetus, particularly related to complications in labour.

During history taking, careful scrutiny of the documentation of the labour and birth is important because there may be factors highlighted that could impact fetal adaption to extrauterine life (Public Health England, 2018) and its natural progression into newborn status. Complications arising in labour that affect fetal oxygenation can be significant and cause long-term effects on neurological development, some of which may be detected by the NIPE practitioner on the first assessment. These may be observed during the assessment of newborn behaviour and the musculoskeletal system, when the normal responses may be absent, exaggerated or outside the expected range of normal, for example lack of muscle tone, absent reflexes and asymmetry in the range of limb movement (Tappero and Honeyfield, 2014).

Equally the mode and type of birth may also have an effect on the neurological and physical complications, such as bruising, cuts and even fractures of bones. This may be significant in women with diabetes who, if the diabetes is not well controlled, have an increased risk of having a macrosomic newborn. Due to the large size this increases the risk of birth injury and perinatal mortality. Injuries may occur due to prolonged labour and shoulder dystocia (NICE, 2015a). Thorough examination of the skeleton around the neck and arms may reveal injuries not always evident on gross examination. Clear documentation of any observed abnormality is essential at this first examination to ensure that appropriate referrals can be made if necessary (Public Health England, 2018).

THINK POINT

What other potential causes could there be for bruising on a newborn's skin?

A key element for the NIPE practitioner to consider is the condition of the newborn immediately after birth. Was any resuscitation required and how well and quickly did the newborn respond to this support? This may give the NIPE practitioner a potential indication of how severe or prolonged an intrapartum hypoxic/anoxic event may have been. The NIPE practitioner should review the labour records rather than the labour summary because this will offer a clear picture of events during the labour and birth (Public Health England, 2016).

Taken together, documentation of the placenta and cord should also be evaluated, taking note of any abnormalities. Immediate cord blood samples obtained at birth will offer the NIPE practitioner an understanding of fetal condition (Malin et al., 2010); these results may support observations during the assessment, particularly if there is any deviation from the normal. Placental health such as grittiness may suggest impact by maternal or environmental factors, such as smoking, drugs or raised blood pressure, all of which will potentially reduce fetal circulation and oxygenation. Placental size is linked to gestation and fetal weight, which may indicate growth restriction if the placenta is smaller than expected. Cord vessels also need to be considered, with the normal configuration of two arteries and one vein generally needed to support normal development, the arteries being directly linked to renal development (Tappero and Honeyfield, 2014). The presence of only one artery may suggest renal agenesis or abnormality, although there may not be any visible signs on external examination; this does require referral and follow-up to ascertain normal internal anatomy (Public Health England, 2018).

CLINICAL TIP

Do not limit yourself to summaries in clinical records, read the notes in full if available as it may provide additional information not immediately evident in a summary.

Postnatal period

At every stage of the childbearing continuum there are influences that can make an impact on fetal/newborn development. Having discussed the early pregnancy/antenatal effects on the developing fetus born to women with complex needs, further consideration is now given to the effects of maternal factors during the postnatal period.

THINK POINT

When would you expect to see physiological jaundice appear in a newborn? What are the current recommendations for the management of physiological jaundice?

Often the first signs of complications due to blood incompatibilities or antibody transmission can be seen early in newborn life, with haemolytic disease causing pathological jaundice presenting within the first 24 hours (Daniels and Bromilow, 2014). The NIPE practitioner's assessment of the skin needs to be thorough and performed in a good light source, to ensure that a comprehensive assessment can be undertaken (see Chapter 6F). Recognition and differentiation of physiological and pathological jaundice is an essential skill for practitioners (Lomax, 2015).

There is further guidance on the recognition and management of physiological jaundice in Chapter 6F.

Once born, maternal smoking, alcohol intake and substance use will continue to have an impact on the newborn. NIPE practitioners are in a unique position to give direct health education during the first assessment; however, care needs to be taken when raising lifestyle changes with the family (Public Health England, 2016). Information can be provided about the effects of smoking and the increased rates of infant mortality (Department of Health, 2017); equally recognition of the signs of neonatal abstinence syndrome (Kocherlakota, 2014) may alert the NIPE practitioner to antenatal substance use not previously revealed during pregnancy, which would require further investigations.

THINK POINT

Are you aware of the signs to look for that may indicate neonatal abstinence syndrome?

Due to the risk factors for babies born to women who are diabetic, communication of information to these women is important. This can prepare the parents for the potential that their infant will be admitted to a neonatal/special care unit for close observation in the early hours after birth. Ultimately the aim is always to keep mother and infant together unless clinically indicated (NICE, 2015). Unlike other newborns, these babies will require additional interventions related to blood glucose monitoring, because this is often affected by maternal circulation during pregnancy. Once born the newborn's ability to regulate his or her own blood glucose will change, with the potential impact of hypoglycaemia if early feeding is not achieved (NICE, 2015; British Association of Perinatal Medicine [BAPM], 2017). As a NIPE practitioner you will need to review the infant's records to establish the type and frequency of feeding since birth, alongside maintenance of normal blood glucose levels. Recommendation for feeding can be more frequent in the early days, which may equate to 2–3 hourly to maintain plasma glucose levels at a minimum of 2.0 mmol/l (NICE, 2015a). For NIPE practitioners it is important to have knowledge of current evidence and local guidance to enable health promotion messages to be given during the NIPE, and to ensure that women are supported to recognise the needs of their infant.

THINK POINT

What are your local trust guidelines in respect of newborn blood glucose monitoring? Take some time to look at the BAPM Identification and Management of Neonatal Hypoglycaemia in the Full Term Infant Framework for Practice (BAPM, 2017).

As previously outlined fetuses of women with epilepsy have the potential to be adversely affected by AEDs during pregnancy. For you as the NIPE practitioner, close observations in the postnatal period and during the NIPE assessment will alert you to potential complications caused by AEDs during *in utero* exposure. Although antenatal exposure does cause a higher incidence of anomalies, current evidence suggests that there is little adverse risk on cognitive development with the transmission of AEDs through breast milk (RCOG, 2016), which is important for you to recognise when providing advice and information on infant feeding.

Throughout this chapter the maternal factors that influence fetal development such as obstetric, medical, social and environmental factors have been discussed. The chapter has focused on key medical conditions that are most commonly seen, for example diabetes and epilepsy. However, there are other conditions that you will need to consider during the NIPE assessment. A general overview of transmittable conditions and viruses has also been included. Further reading on transmittable diseases would be recommended to support knowledge to help you as a NIPE practitioner. The chapter included a brief introduction to some areas of NIPE assessment, many of which are covered in more detail within the guide.

References

British Association of Perinatal Medicine (2017). *Identification and Management of Neonatal Hypoglycaemia in the Full Term Infant Framework for Practice*. Available at: www.bapm.org/resources/identification-and-management-neonatal-hypoglycaemia-full-term-infant-%E2%80%93-framework-practice (accessed 14 November 2018).

Behnke, M. and Smith, V.C. (2013). Prenatal substance abuse: short- and long-term effects on the exposed fetus. *Pediatrics*, **131**: 1009–24.

Cleft Lip and Palate Association (n.d.) What is cleft lip and palate? Available at: www.clapa.com/what-is-cleft-lip-palate (accessed 20 April 2018).

Coton, S.J., Nazareth, I. and Petersen, I. (2016). A cohort study of trends in the prevalence of pregestational diabetes in pregnancy recorded in UK general practice between 1995 and 2012. *BMJ Open* **6**: e009494.

Daniels, G. and Bromilow, I. (2014). *Essential Guide to Blood Groups*, 3rd edn. Chichester: Wiley Blackwell.

Department of Health (2016). *UK Chief Medical Officers' Low Risk Drinking Guidelines*. London: DH. Available at: www.gov.uk/government/publications/alcohol-consumption-advice-on-low-risk-drinking (accessed 10 April 2018).

Department of Health (2017). Mothers and Babies Reducing Risk through Audit and Confidential Enquires across the UK (MBRRACE-UK). *Perinatal Confidential Enquiry – Term, Singleton, Intrapartum Stillbirth and Intrapartum Related Neonatal Death*. Leicester: DH.

Kocherlakota, P. (2014). Neonatal abstinence syndrome. *Pediatrics*, **134**: 547–61.

Lomax, A. (2015). *Examination of the Newborn: An Evidence-Based Guide*, 2nd edn. Chichester: Wiley Blackwell.

Malin, G.L., Morris, R.K. and Khan, K.S. (2010). Strength of association between umbilical cord pH and perinatal and long term outcomes: Systematic review and meta-analysis. *BJM Online* 1–13.

National Institute for Health and Care Excellence (NICE) (2010). *Pregnancy and Complex Social Factors: A model for service provision for women with complex social factors*. London: NICE.

National Institute for Health and Care Excellence (2014). *Hepatitis B*. London: NICE.

National Institute for Health and Care Excellence (2015a). *Diabetes in Pregnancy: Management from preconception to the postnatal period*. London: NICE.

National Institute for Health and Care Excellence (2015b). *Antenatal Care for Uncomplicated Pregnancies*. London: NICE.

Public Health England (2016). *Newborn and Infant Physical Examination Screening Programme Standards 2016/17*. Available at: www.gov.uk/government/uploads/system/uploads/attachment_data/file/524424/NIPE_Programme_Standards_2016_to_2017.pdf (accessed 20 April 2018),

Public Health England (2018). *Newborn and Infant Physical Examination Programme Handbook*. Available at: www.gov.uk/government/publications/newborn-and-infant-physical-examination-programme-handbook/newborn-and-infant-physical-examination-screening-programme-handbook (accessed 19 April 2018).

Royal College of Obstetrics and Gynaecology (RCOG) (2010). *Greentop Guidelines No. 39: Management of HIV in Pregnancy*. London: RCOG.

Royal College of Obstetrics and Gynaecology (2015). *Greentop Guidelines No. 13: Chicken Pox in Pregnancy*. London: RCOG.

Royal College of Obstetrics and Gynaecology (2016). *Greentop Guidelines No. 68: Epilepsy in Pregnancy*. London: RCOG.

Sadler, T.W. (2015). *Langman's Medical Embryology*, 13th edn. Philadelphia, PA: Wolters Kluwer.

Tappero, E.P. and Honeyfield, M.E. (2014). *Physical Assessment of the Newborn: A Comprehensive Approach to the Art of Physical Examination*, 5th edn. New York: Springer.

5 Why the maternal history is important for the NIPE practitioner in performing a safe and through examination

Kim Wilcock

Introduction

This chapter focuses on the importance of obtaining a detailed, accurate and factual history before undertaking the newborn infant physical examination (NIPE). Obtaining a comprehensive history underpins the NIPE and can help the practitioner distinguish infants who are deemed low risk and therefore eligible to be examined under your sphere of practice. Moreover, a thorough examination of the history can identify infants who may require timely referral to specialist services. Emphasis is placed on how to undertake a systematic approach during history taking and guidance on where to look to retrieve relevant clinical records. Furthermore, this chapter discusses why reviewing antepartum, intrapartum and the immediate postpartum history is important, and why possible interventions and screening have taken place throughout pregnancy and the relevance of those results in relation to the NIPE.

Preceding physical examination, it is vital for NIPE practitioners to obtain accurate and factual information (Public Health England, 2018). The documented history taken during booking appointments, the admission and routine assessment enables practitioners to assess risk and refer deviations appropriately. As a NIPE practitioner, examination of the pregnancy history will broaden your understanding of the environment that the fetus has occupied during the childbearing continuum, making the examination specific to that family and infant (Public Health England, 2018; UK National Screening Committee, 2017). Vigilance is sought when reviewing clinical documentation to make use of the valuable information that is available and accessible in clinical maternal records (Medical Research Council, 2018). This chapter will help you to understand what information might be available and useful for the NIPE.

Due to the busy nature of the clinical setting and potential distractions, it is important that the practitioner finds a quiet location to review the records. It is also important to allow adequate time to review all elements of the maternal and newborn history, avoiding distractions from colleagues, patients or visitors where possible. Distractions may result in the practitioner missing a step in the history process, resulting in suboptimal practice and missed opportunities to identify abnormalities in a timely manner. Early identification of at-risk neonates and subsequent management have been shown to reduce morbidity and mortality rates (British Association of Perinatal Medicine, 2015). Clinical proformas (Figure 5.1) and questionnaires can help to eliminate this risk by structuring the process and providing the opportunity to re-visit maternal history. Discussion with the family would complete the history-taking process, allowing appropriate questioning and exploration of any findings.

A three-step approach to history taking is considered:

Step 1: use a proforma to structure the history-taking process (Figure 5.1).

Step 2: provide a questionnaire for parents to complete asking specific questions relating to maternal health and wellbeing, family history of congenital abnormalities or metabolic disorders, and immediate neonatal history including feeding, elimination and any concerns that they might have.

Step 3: re-visit important questions relating to maternal and neonatal history, parental lifestyle habits or parental concerns.

Step 1

History-taking proformas (see Figure 5.1) have been designed to enable practitioners to obtain a thorough history by following a systematic approach. Typically, NIPE history proformas prompt retrieval of information from expected date of delivery (EDD), serological results and the booking history, to intrapartum details, postnatal observations and early newborn behaviour. The practitioner would follow each section and document the findings accordingly. Proformas guide the process and may prevent the practitioner from missing an important step in the history taking.

Step 2

Providing questionnaires for families to complete before undertaking the NIPE will allow the NIPE practitioner to re-visit questions with families including; maternal health and wellbeing, medication, family history, congenital abnormalities and relevant health of any siblings. Through these questionnaires, families are encouraged to document feeding history, elimination

NEWBORN HISTORY FORM

Date...

Name.. D.O.B...

BIRTH HISTORY

Was your infant full term?.............. Pre-term?.................. Adopted?........................

If pre-term, how many weeks?.................. If adopted at what age?........................

Type of delivery Vaginal.................... C-Section............................

If C-Section please explain why...

Please describe any problems after birth..

Where there any problems during pregnancy?..

Was your infant exposed to tobacco, alcohol or drugs during pregnancy?...............................

Did your infant pass the hearing screen in the hospital? Yes........................ No...............................

Did your infant have a newborn blood spot test/metabolic screen completed? Yes...
No...................................

Was your infant Breech any time in thee last month of pregnancy? Yes............... No................

FAMILY HISTORY

Do any family members have any of the following conditions?

Condition	Mother	Father	Sibling	Grandparent
High Blood Pressure				
High Cholesterol				
Prolonged QT				
Early Heart Attack (Under 50 years)				
Sudden Unexplained Death				
Anaemia				
Bleeding or Clotting Disorder				
Allergies				
Autoimmune Disorder				
Cancer				
Genetic Disease				
Diabetes				
Thyroid Disease				
Polycystic Ovary Syndrome				

Figure 5.1
Example of a newborn history form

history and behaviour of the newborn, and, lastly, highlight any concerns that the parents may have regarding their infant.

Step 3

Discussion with the family enables practitioners to ask questions relating to maternal or family history. This will also provide the opportunity to offer health promotion advice, make any referrals to specialist services and offer an opportunity for any parental concerns to be addressed. Thorough discussion with the mother and family is important to strengthen the quality of the history profile. Ideally both parents should be present during the history-taking discussion to obtain as thorough a history profile as possible.

The art of history taking requires sensitivity and trust, which is an important skill to develop: maintaining open body language, keeping eye contact and listening, and showing empathy, kindness and compassion are vital for effective communication (Nursing Midwifery Council, 2015) (see Chapter 3). Appropriate, relevant questioning must be specific to each individual family, ensuring that questions are culturally appropriate and suitable for women who do not speak or read English. It might be that this approach needs to be altered according to the needs of the family should they have additional physical, sensory or learning needs (National Institute for Care Excellence [NICE], 2017). The NIPE practitioner's awareness of the woman's history will strengthen the NIPE and prepare them for potential questions surrounding sensitive topics, for example previous stillbirth, neonatal death or sudden infant death. The skilled practitioner will adapt the examination to address the specific family concerns appropriately, particularly if they have had concerns relating to any screening results.

The booking exam and antenatal care

The aim of antenatal care is to monitor the health of the mother and fetus, screen for potential abnormalities, and provide information and education to the mother and family in preparation for parenthood (NICE, 2010a). This is important for the NIPE practitioner to recognise because fetal development and wellbeing can be influenced by events that take place during the childbearing continuum (Sadler, 2015). As discussed in Chapter 4, obstetric, medical, psychosocial and environmental factors can influence fetal development. The booking appointment and subsequent antenatal care risk assess maternal and family history, and offer appropriate screening, education and interventions to minimise risks during the childbearing continuum. According to NICE (2010c) this should take place by 10 weeks' gestation, so that appropriate screening and interventions can be offered in a timely manner. The booking appointment, screening investigations and subsequent antenatal care can provide vital information relating to the NIPE practitioner, and each is considered in turn.

> ## CLINICAL TIP
>
> The booking appointment will provide the following information:
>
> - Maternal health and wellbeing during current and previous pregnancies
> - Maternal surgical and medical history
> - Family traits and congenital abnormalities.

Sensitivity should be sought during history taking if the family have had assisted conception; with donor eggs or sperm there may in this instance be limited information available about the genetic background.

> ## THINK POINT
>
> Consider how maternal age can have a potential impact on the fetus.

Age-related congenital conditions are associated with advancing maternal age and teenage pregnancies (Department of Health, 2017a). Teenage pregnancy is associated with poorer perinatal outcomes and a greater need for health promotion and education (Public Health England, 2016a). Advancing maternal age is correspondingly related to poorer outcomes. There is an association with advancing maternal age in relation to infertility problems and raised body mass index (BMI), which is also associated with pregnancy complications such as gestational diabetes, hypertension, venous thromboembolism, macrosomia, shoulder dystocia and subsequent neonatal hypoglycaemia (Department of Health, 2017a).

Pregnancy-related complications such as: pre-eclampsia, eclampsia, HELLP (haemolysis, elevated liver enzymes, low platelets), venous thromboembolism and gestational diabetes must be appreciated when compiling the history profile of the mother. Mild or moderate gestational hypertension increases the risk of growth restriction due to placental disease; subsequently infants are at risk of being small for gestational age, usually measuring below the 10th centile or being born preterm. Ultrasound is indicated for fetal growth, amniotic fluid volume and umbilical artery Doppler velocimetry (NICE, 2010b). Accessing additional investigations, such as ultrasound, affords the opportunity to forewarn the practitioner of potential newborn complications. Previous obstetric history can also provide vital information relating to the health of siblings. Previous pregnancies with poor outcomes, for example intrauterine death or sudden infant death syndrome (SIDS), may involve follow-up investigations or referral.

> ## THINK POINT
>
> Do you know what resources are available to support families who have a history of SIDS? Look at your trust guidance and resources. Do you sign-post parents to external organisations?

Practitioners should be alert to family traits because they carry an inherited risk for the newborn. Any known genetic disorders must be noted and explored due to the risk of inheritance (see Chapter 7). The significance of congenital abnormalities, such as congenital heart disease in a first-degree relative or sibling, carries a recurrence risk of 2–3% for the newborn, or 5% if the newborn's parents have congenital heart disease (Tappero and Honeyfield, 2014; Public Health England, 2018). In this instance, it would be appropriate for the NIPE examination to be completed by a member of the medical team. Family history may also reveal risk factors associated with developmental dysplasia of the hip (DDH) if a first-degree family member reports childhood hip problems. A congenital history of hereditary cataracts (first-degree relative) and exposure to viruses during pregnancy, including rubella and cytomegalovirus, are areas of importance and need to be considered if highlighted. Cryptorchidism affects 2–6% of male babies and increases the risk of testicular cancer and reduced fertility; associated risk factors include: first-degree family history of cryptorchidism; having this information can assist with a thorough examination but all male infants should have their testes examined as part of the screen (see Chapter 6) (Public Health England, 2018).

> ## THINK POINT
>
> A family trait is an inherited genetic likeness. Explore some common genetic disorders that can impact on the health of the newborn (see Chapter 7).

Family history may raise cultural practices; the experienced NIPE practitioner must be prepared for this situation. It is important to establish whether parents share relatives due to the risks of autosomal and recessive conditions. Female genital mutilation (FGM) is practised in many countries, including Africa, Asia and the Middle East. Healthcare professionals have a responsibility to safeguard the public (NMC, 2015), because this practice is illegal in the UK. If FGM has been disclosed during pregnancy and the newborn is female, she may be at risk; the practitioner must be alert to the safeguarding implications surrounding FGM and be clear of the trust child protection guidance or know who to contact for further guidance (Department of Health, 2017b). Sharing information with multi-agency partners and local safeguarding leads may allow interventions to be put in place, thereby protecting the newborn from FGM in the future. NIPE practitioners have a responsibility to raise concerns if any safeguarding issues are identified.

CLINICAL TIP

Make yourself aware of the trust safeguarding guidance and key professionals.

The effects of domestic abuse on children's social, emotional, psychological and educational wellbeing are well known (NICE, 2014b). Knowledge of local guidelines, safeguarding leads and appropriate referral pathways initiates early intervention. Raised awareness and vigilance during history taking and subsequent interaction with the family may alert you, as the NIPE practitioner, to an abusive relationship. Domestic abuse is also linked to mental ill health and adverse lifestyle choices, including smoking, alcohol and substance misuse (NICE, 2014b). Adverse lifestyle choices are well known to have a direct impact on fetal wellbeing. Smoking, alcohol and substance misuse are associated with co-morbidities, poor fetal growth, preterm delivery and newborn anomalies, and increased mortality (Behnke and Smith, 2013; Sadler, 2015).

THINK POINT

If you suspected domestic abuse, consider how you would approach the subject. Discuss this with your mentor.

In this instance, accessing support from the safeguarding midwife or child protection team will equip you with the strategies to approach the situation safely and sensitively. The maternal history can be a wealth of information for the NIPE practitioner, helping you to be prepared.

As previously outlined, screening investigations are implemented to detect abnormalities. Ultrasound scanning can identify neural tube defects, talipes or structural defects, and serological screening identifies increased risks of inherited disorders such as sickle-cell anaemia and thalassaemia, or infections such as human immunodeficiency virus (HIV), hepatitis B or syphilis. Early ultrasound scanning is recommended between 10 weeks 0 days and 13 weeks 6 days to determine gestational age. This is then followed by ultrasound screening for fetal anomalies between 18 weeks 0 days and 20 weeks 6 days (NICE, 2017). Serological information can provide information on the wellbeing of the mother or any treatment provided, for example anaemia. Screening for anaemia, sickle-cell and thalassaemia, blood group and rhesus D status takes place during the booking appointment and at 28 weeks. It is recommended that routine antenatal anti-D prophylaxis be offered to all non-sensitised pregnant women who are rhesus D negative. Blood group and rhesus factor predisposing to incompatibility can cause haemolytic disease in the newborn. NIPE practitioners should explore results from all serological investigations to identify newborns at risk of inherited traits or infections. Hepatitis B screening may identify a positive result; in this instance, the newborn may require vaccination with hepatitis B immune globulin (HBIG) and follow-up care (NICE, 2014a).

Serological investigations are offered to screen for the genetic disorder trisomy 21 known as Down's syndrome. The 'combined test' (nuchal translucency, β-human chorionic gonadotrophin, pregnancy-associated plasma protein-A) is offered at 11 weeks 0 days and 13 weeks 6 days, or a triple or quadruple test between 15 weeks 0 days and 20 weeks 0 days (NICE, 2010a). Results may have identified an increased risk during pregnancy; practitioners should be alert to the potential risks before physical examination. Parents may be particularly anxious, so the role of the NIPE practitioner would be to draw attention to normal findings during the assessment.

THINK POINT

Screening for Down's syndrome indicates a high-risk result. What characteristics would you be looking for during the NIPE? See Chapter 7 for further information.

Ongoing antenatal care will inform practitioners of the health and wellbeing of the mother and fetus during the antepartum period. Blood pressure measurements and urinalysis for protein are carried out at each antenatal visit to screen for pre-eclampsia. Symphysis–fundal height is measured and recorded at each antenatal appointment from 24 weeks for growth. Fetal presentation is assessed by abdominal palpation at 36 weeks and could provide important information if the fetus is presenting as breech. Under current guidance, nulliparous women with an uncomplicated pregnancy are schedule 10 appointments with 7 appointments offered to parous women (NICE, 2017). Table 5.1 Provides a checklist of information retrieved from the booking appointment and antenatal care; this list forms the basis of the history profile, looking at maternal and fetal health and wellbeing, past and present obstetric history, maternal medical and family history, psychosocial influences and medication. Table 5.2 presents the routine serological investigations recommended by NICE.

THINK POINT

Start to compile your own history profile checklist. Table 5.1 provides some examples of booking history and antenatal information relevant to the NIPE.

Table 5.1 Checklist of information retrieved from the booking appointment	
Booking/antenatal documentation	Relevance to the NIPE
Last menstrual period (LMP) Expected date of delivery (EDD)	Gestational age assessment
Parity/past obstetric history	Hearing impairments, cardiac abnormalities, developmental dysplasia of the hips, hereditary eye conditions Additional support needs of siblings Infection, previous stillbirth, SID, neonatal death
Ethnicity	Some genetic disorders are more prevalent, for example sickle-cell anaemia
Maternal paternal and family information	Family traits Family history of exposure to active tuberculosis Cardiac (family history of congenital heart disease (first-degree relative) Hips: first-degree family history of hip problems during childhood or as an infant Eyes: history includes: family history of congenital or hereditary cataracts (first-degree relative) Testes: first-degree family history of cryptorchidism
Maternal sociodemographic information	Maternal age (teenagers or women over 40 higher risk of complications) Women particularly vulnerable or lacking support Obesity or underweight BMI
Maternal general health including pre-existing conditions, medical and surgical history	Infertility Cardiac disease including hypertension Renal disease Endocrine disorders Diabetes Hypothyroidism Haematological disorders Autoimmune disorders, Epilepsy Malignant disease Severe asthma
Psychosocial influences	Domestic abuse Smoking Intravenous drug users Substance use: cannabis, heroin, cocaine (including crack cocaine) and Ecstasy Alcohol dependency Depression

Table 5.1 Continued

Ultrasound scans and investigations	Gestational age scan Fetal anomaly scan (structural anomalies) Soft markers Nuchal translucency Chorionic villous sampling Amniocentesis
Maternal wellbeing during current pregnancy	Supplementation with vitamin D Folic acid Anaemia Listeriosis and salmonella infection, toxoplasmosis Maternal exposure to viruses in pregnancy including rubella and cytomegalovirus Travelling abroad during pregnancy Hypertension, gestational hypertension, pre-eclampsia, eclampsia, HELLP Venous thromboembolism, gestational diabetes, epilepsy, systemic lupus erythematosus Past or present depression, severe mental illness or psychiatric treatment Rh sensitisation
Fetal wellbeing during current pregnancy	Poor fetal growth (review customised growth chart) Polyhydramnios (oesophageal atresia), oligohydramnios and wellbeing during the antenatal period Small for gestational age (below 5th centile) Large for gestational age (above 95th centile)
Safeguarding/child protection	Female genital mutilation Domestic abuse Safeguarding issues/social worker involvement
Medication	Anticonvulsant drugs Analgesia Antidepressants Antiepileptic drugs Anticoagulants Antihypertensives Sedatives and psychiatric drugs

Table 5.2 Serological investigations

Screening

Blood group and rhesus D status	Blood group and red-cell alloantibodies (including prophylaxis with anti-D)
Complete blood count	Haemoglobin
Haemoglobinopathies	Thalassaemia or sickle-cell anaemia Screening for haematological conditions: sickle-cell anaemia and thalassaemia
Disease/Infection	Rubella Chlamydia infection Syphilis Hepatitis B Hepatitis C HIV
Combined test	Nuchal translucency, β-human chorionic gonadotrophin, pregnancy-associated plasma protein-A
Triple or quadruple test (Down's syndrome screening)	Triple or quadruple test screening for Down's syndrome
Additional serology screening (not offered as routine screening)	Group B streptococci Kleihauer–Betke test Toxoplasmosis

Intrapartum

Retrieving a comprehensive intrapartum history will highlight potential risk factors for the newborn, promote vigilance for potential abnormalities and prepare practitioners for parental concerns and questions. Taking account of the intrapartum journey also affords the opportunity to verify appropriate newborn aftercare, investigations and referral. Having knowledge of the length of labour, analgesia, presentation, position and mode of delivery will make you vigilant to potential birth injuries and trauma (Table 5.3). Caput succedaneum, excessive moulding, cephalhaematoma and scalp injuries are associated with long labours, malposition and instrumental births (Whitby et al., 2004; O'Mahoney et al., 2010). Breech presentation at or after 36 weeks' gestation in a singleton, or twins if one is breech, requires referral for ultrasound of the hips (see Chapter 6E). According to the UK NSC (Public Health England, 2016b) ultrasound should be performed on both babies (of the twins) before age 6 weeks. This is due to the difficulty in identifying which infant may have been affected.

THINK POINT

Analgesia or anaesthesia administered during the intrapartum period can affect feeding and behaviour and cause respiratory depression due to the adverse effect on the respiratory system.

Do you know which drugs cross the placenta and the potential side effects on the newborn?

Group B haemolytic *Streptococcus* (GBS) is associated with increased mortality rates due to the correlation between GBS and early onset group B *Streptococcus* (EOGBS) in the neonate. Routine screening is not, however, recommended in the UK (UK NSC, 2017).

Infection status and history

Colonised mothers are offered intrapartum antibiotic prophylaxis (IAP) to reduce the incidence of EOGBS disease (NICE, 2012; Royal College of Obstetricians and Gynaecologists [RCOG], 2017). A Cochrane review identified reduced incidence of EOGBS with IAP (relative risk 0.14; 95% confidence interval [CI] 0.04–0.74) in colonised mothers; the numbers of deaths were too small to assess the impact on mortality (Ohlsson and Shah, 2014). NIPE practitioners should be alert to risk factors associated with EOGBS, including: previous infant with GBS, maternal GBS carriage during pregnancy, identified by bacterial investigation, preterm birth, prolonged rupture of the membranes, pyrexia or suspected maternal intrapartum infection (RCOG, 2017). Maternal temperature of 38.6°C or ruptured membranes for more than 24 hours are associated with an increased risk of EOGBS (NICE, 2012; RCOG, 2017); local policy may indicate investigations including obtaining swabs from the newborn to rule out infection. Local guidance might also include carrying out newborn vital signs for 12 hours; you could use the Newborn Early Warning scoring system (BAPM, 2015). NIPE history taking should include appraisal of maternal intrapartum details to establish administration of IAP and appropriate aftercare for the newborn. The recommended action for women who decline IAP is close observation of the newborn's vital signs for 12 hours; antibiotic treatment may be required if there are clinical signs of EOGBS disease (RCOG, 2017).

CLINICAL TIP

Check intrapartum documentation for: preterm birth, prolonged rupture of the membranes, pyrexia or suspected maternal intrapartum infection. Look for maternal investigations for GBS colonisation. Observe dating scan and the last menstrual period for preterm birth. Confirm IAP administration and, if indicated, that newborn vital signs have been completed and are within normal parameters.

THINK POINT

It is important to alert families to the signs of potential EOGBS.

What advice would you give to parents to look for signs of EOGBS in the newborn?

Meconium-stained liquor would alert the practitioner to verify documentation for appropriate newborn aftercare, and confirm that vital signs are within normal parameters. If there are risk factors that meconium was passed before or during labour then this has the potential to cause infection and increased risk of meconium aspiration syndrome (NICE, 2014b). This condition can result in severe respiratory difficulties requiring neonatal unit admission. NICE (2014b) endorse close observation and vital signs in the presence of significant meconium for the first 12 hours, and 2 hours for non-significant meconium.

THINK POINT

It is important to alert families to the signs of infection.

Make a note of what vital signs should be observed in the newborn in the presence of meconium-stained liquor and what advice could be given to parents.

Documentation of obstetric emergencies during the intrapartum period would prompt the NIPE practitioner to review maternal documentation closely and consider further screening due to the risk of hypoxia. In the event of a cord prolapse, suboptimal cardiotocograph, acute antepartum/intrapartum haemorrhage or fetal bradycardia, cord bloods would provide valuable information on the condition of the newborn immediately after birth.

Birth injuries

Following recognition of a shoulder dystocia, the NIPE practitioner should check the birth records to ensure a paediatrician has examined the newborn after delivery or pre-empt the need for a more thorough check of the clavicles or referral for a radiograph. Fetal injuries associated with shoulder dystocia include: fractures of the humerus and clavicle, pneumothoraces and hypoxic brain injury (Ouzounian et al., 1997; Gherman et al., 1998). Brachial plexus injury has been reported in 2.3–16% of instances of shoulder dystocia (Draycott et al., 2008; Gherman et al., 1997, 1998). Obstetric emergency follow-up care for the newborn is often stipulated locally or in accordance with national guidelines. NIPE practitioners should be alert to additional information

including: resuscitation of the newborn, Apgar scores, vital signs and hypoglycaemia guidelines.

CLINICAL TIP

Check your local guidelines to familiarise yourself with neonatal aftercare
after obstetric emergency.

Table 5.3 Intrapartum history

Mode of birth: Normal birth, instrumental or operative birth	Birth injury and trauma Condition at birth

Presentation:
Cephalic, breech
	Breech presentation at 36 weeks or
	    birth requires ultrasound follow-up
	    referral

Date and time of birth	Appropriate timescales to perform
	    NIPE, adaptation to extrauterine life
	    (heart murmurs common in the first
	    24 hours)

First and second stage length	Condition of infant (excessive
	    moulding, caput), precipitate birth
	    (facial congestion and risk of
	    tentorial tear)

Complications during labour	Group B Strep (appropriate plans
	    should be made before birth in
	    response to anticipated risk factors)
	Liquor (meconium present or
	    offensive liquor)
	Temperature during labour
	Time of ruptured membranes (history
	    of PROM)

Complications	Birth trauma, shoulder dystocia
	Cord vessels checked
	Placenta and cord abnormalities
	Cord bloods (arterial, venous; blood
	    group rhesus; Coombs' test and
	    antibodies)
	Apgar score
	Neonatal resuscitation

Analgesia, anaesthesia and other drugs administered and times if relevant	Opiates General anaesthetic Antihypertensives Magnesium sulphate

Completion of the intrapartum history would involve the practitioner noting the condition of the placenta and cord vessels. Practitioners should confirm that two arteries and one vein have been documented. A single artery is associated with renal abnormalities, Potters' syndrome or Edwards' syndrome (trisomy 18).

THINK POINT

Can you think of any conditions associated with a large placenta? Discuss this with your mentor.

Postpartum

Postnatal records contain valuable information on the condition of the newborn at birth and the early postnatal period (see Table 5.3). Apgar scores, venous and arterial cord blood results (if available), and the extent of any resuscitation that was required facilitate an understanding of the condition of the newborn immediately after birth, including any associated risks of hypothermia and hypoglycaemia. A thorough history profile will require you, as the NIPE practitioner, gaining access to any additional investigations that have been reported. To reiterate, the presence of meconium-stained liquor (NICE, 2014b), GBS-colonised mothers (RCOG, 2017), resuscitation of the newborn or low cord pH results (Malin et al., 2010) all assist you in gathering an overview of any abnormal findings that need to be considered. NIPE practitioners must also be vigilant for infants born to mothers with diabetes or gestational diabetes, and observe blood glucose monitoring results according to their trust's guidelines (NICE, 2015; BAPM, 2017). Serological investigations, for example serum bilirubin investigations for jaundice (NICE, 2010b), could also be noted, so you must confirm that results have been documented and are within normal parameters.

Parental information

New parents scrutinise their newborn and may have observed physical or behavioural features or signs and symptoms; during your interaction this information is important for you as a NIPE practitioner. Encourage the woman and her family to discuss any concerns – physical, social, mental or emotional – that they might have (NICE, 2006). Documentation will provide evidence of newborn behaviour, feeding methods and frequency, and passage of meconium and urine. It is good clinical practice to enhance the quality of the information by having a discussion with the mother and family about these factors, encouraging expression of any questions or concerns. Newborn behaviour, feeding and elimination emphasise the status of the neurological and gastrointestinal systems.

CLINICAL TIP

Useful things to ask families:

Information related to feeding and elimination

Time of first feed

Method of feeding and frequency

Passage of meconium or urine (urine stream in a boy)

Newborn behaviour: does the newborn wake for feeds? Is the newborn alert and well and showing good tone or is he or she sleepy or restless?

It is important to practise within professional boundaries and sphere of practice (NMC, 2015) and according to trust guidance; it is also important that you have access to individual trust guidance about the NIPE role and an understanding of your responsibility as a NIPE practitioner. You need to be aware of referral pathways and limitations within your role when undertaking NIPE examinations. Public Health England's (2017) *Newborn and Infant Physical Examination, Service Specification*, the *NIPE Screening Programme Standards* (Public Health England, 2016b) and the *NIPE Programme Handbook* (Public Health

Table 5.4 Postnatal history

Birth weight	<2.5 kg or >4.5 kg and head circumference on growth chart
Infant records	Vital signs, behaviour and individual postnatal plans Check passed meconium and urine (urine stream in a boy) Vitamin K (dose/route) Method of feeding concerns, time of first feed
Establish any parental/carer anxieties	Parental concerns or observations
Congenital abnormality	Structural or chromosomal
Hearing	Hearing screening completed/referral
Serological investigations	Blood group Infection screening Serum bilirubin
Immunisation	Hepatitis B BCG (Bacille Calmette–Guérin)

England, 2018) support best clinical practice and should be used to underpin NIPE history taking.

> ## CLINICAL TIP
>
> Ensure that you are familiar with local policy surrounding your sphere of practice in undertaking the NIPE, specifically any infants deemed to require a NIPE by a medical practitioner.

Throughout this chapter the importance of obtaining a detailed, accurate, factual history has been explored. Practitioners are signposted to antepartum, intrapartum and postpartum documentation, and their relevance to NIPE. Clinical tips and think boxes have been provided to help you expand your knowledge and encourage further reading. An overview has been provided exploring many factors relevant to NIPE. The booking appointment, serological results, screening, intrapartum records and early neonatal period have been explored throughout.

References

Behnke, M. and Smith, V.C. (2013). Prenatal substance abuse: short- and long-term effects on the exposed fetus. *Pediatrics*, **131**(3): 1009–24.

British Association of Perinatal Medicine (2015). *Newborn Early Warning Track and Trigger (NEWTT): A Framework for Practice*. Available at: www.bapm.org/publications/documents/guidelines/NEWTT%20framework%20final%20for%20websitepdf (accessed: 23 March 2018).

British Association of Perinatal Medicine (2017). *Identification and Management of Neonatal Hypoglycaemia in the Full Term Infant – A Framework for Practice*. Available at: www.bapm.org/sites/default/files/files/Identification%20and%20Management%20of%20Neonatal%20Hypoglycaemia%20in%20the%20%20full%20term%20infant%20-%20A%20Framework%20for%20Practice%20revised%20Oct%202017.pdf (accessed 30/ October 2018).

Department of Health (2017a). *Mothers and Babies Reducing Risk through Audit and Confidential Enquires across the UK (MBRRACE):UK Perinatal Confidential Enquiry. Term, Singleton, Intrapartum stillbirth and intrapartum-related neonatal death*. Available at: www.npeu.ox.ac.uk/mbrrace-uk/reports (accessed 30 April 2018).

Department of Health (2017b). *FGM Safeguarding and Risk Assessment. Quick Guide for Health Professionals*. London: DH.

Draycott, T.J., Crofts, J.F., Ash, J.P., Wilson, I.V., Yard, E., Sibanda, T. and Whitelaw, A. (2008). Improving neonatal outcome through practical shoulder dystocia training. *Obstetrics and Gynaecology*. **112**: 14–20.

Gherman, R.B., Goodwin, T.M., Souter, I., Neumann, K., Ouzounian, J.G. and Paul, R.H. (1997). The McRoberts' manoeuvre for the alleviation of shoulder dystocia: How successful is it? *American Journal of Obstetrics and Gynecology*, **176**: 656–61.

Gherman, R.B., Ouzounian, J.G., Goodwin, T.M. (1998). Obstetric manoeuvres for shoulder dystocia and associated fetal morbidity. *American Journal of Obstetrics and Gynecology*, **178**: 112–30.

Malin, G.L., Morris, R.K. and Khan, K.S. (2010). Strength of association between umbilical cord pH and perinatal and long-term outcomes: systematic review and meta-analysis. *BJM Online* 1–13.

Medical Research Council (2018). *Sharing Patient Records can Help Researchers Save an Improve Lives.* Available at: www.mrc.ukri.org (accessed 10 September 2018).

National Institute for Health and Care Excellence (NICE) (2006). *Postnatal Care up to 8 Weeks after Birth. NICE Clinical Guideline 37.* Available at: www.nice.org.uk/ guidance/cg37/chapter/1-Recommendations (accessed 25 April 2019).

National Institute for Health and Care Excellence (2010a). *Antenatal Care for Uncomplicated Pregnancies. NICE Clinical Guideline 62.* London: NICE.

National Institute of Health Care and Excellence (2010b). *Jaundice in Newborn Babies under 28 Days. NICE Clinical Guideline 98.* London: NICE.

National Institute of Health Care and Excellence (2010c). Pregnancy and complex social factors: a model for service provision for pregnant women with complex social factors. Available at: www.nice.org.uk/guidance/cg110/chapter/1-Guidance (accessed 25 April 2019).

National Institute of Health Care and Excellence (2012). *Neonatal Infection (Early Onset): Antibiotics for Prevention and Treatment. NICE Clinical Guideline 149.* London: NICE.

National Institute for Health and Clinical Excellence (2014a). *Hepatitis B.* London: NICE.

National Institute of Health Care and Excellence (2014b). *Domestic Violence and Abuse: Multi-agency working. NICE Clinical Guideline PH 50.* London: NICE.

National Institute for Health and Care Excellence (2015). *Diabetes in Pregnancy: Management from preconception to the postnatal period.* London: NICE.

National Institute for Health and Care Excellence (2017). *Antenatal Care for Uncomplicated Pregnancies.* London: NICE.

Nursing and Midwifery Council (NMC) (2015). *The Code: Professional standards of practice and behaviour for nurses and midwives.* London: NMC.

Ohlsson, A. and Shah V.S. (2014). Intrapartum antibiotics for known maternal Group B streptococcal colonization. *Cochrane Database Systematic Review*, 6: CD007467.

O'Mahoney, F., Hofmeyr, G.J. and Menon, V. (2010). Choice of instruments for assisted vaginal delivery. *Cochrane Database of Systematic Review* Available at: http://cochranelibrary-wiley.com/doi/10.1002/14651858.CD005455.pub2/full (accessed: 27 August 2018).

Ouzounian, J.G., Korst, L.M and Phelan, J.P. (1997). Permanent Erb's palsy: A traction related injury? *Obstetrics and Gynaecology*, **89**: 139–41.

Public Health England (2016a). *Teenage Mothers and Young Fathers: Support framework,* May. Available at: www.gov.uk/government/publications/teenage-mothers-and-young-fathers-support-framework (accessed 30 April 2018).

Public Health England (2016b). *Newborn and Infant Physical Examination Screening Programme Standards* 2016/17, April. Available at: www.gov.uk/government/ uploads/system/uploads/attachment_data/file/524424/NIPE_Programme_Standards_2016_to_2017.pdf (accessed 20 April 2018).

Public Health England (2017). *NHS Public Health functions agreement 2017–18. Service Specification No. 21, NHS Newborn and Infant Physical Examination Screening Programme.* Available at: www.england.nhs.uk/wp-content/uploads/2017/06/service-specification-21.pdf (accessed 30 April 2018).

Public Health England (2018). *Newborn and Infant Physical Examination Programme Handbook.* Available at: www.gov.uk/government/publications/newborn-and-infant-physical-examination-programme-handbook/newborn-and-infant-physical-examination-screening-programme-handbook (accessed 19 April 2018).

Royal College of Obstetrics and Gynaecology (RCOG) (2017). *Greentop Guideline 36: The Prevention of Early-onset Neonatal Group B Streptococcal Disease.* London: RCOG.

Sadler, T.W. (2015). *Langman's Medical Embryology*, 13th edn. Philadelphia, PA: Wolters Kluwer.

Tappero, E.P. and Honeyfield, M.E. (2014). *Physical Assessment of the Newborn: A Comprehensive Approach to the Art of Physical Examination*, 5th edn. New York: Springer.

UK National Screening Committee (UK NSC) (2017). *UK NSC Group B Streptococcus (GBS) Recommendation.* London: UK NSC.

Whitby, E.H., Griffiths, P.D., Rutter, S., Smith, M.F., Sprigg, A., Ohadike, P. et al. (2004). Frequency and natural history of subdural haemorrhages in babies and relation to obstetric factors. *Lancet*, **68**(363): 846–51.

6 The physical examination

A step-by-step approach

Tracey Jones

This chapter covers the physical examination using a step-by-step approach. Any practitioner carrying out the newborn infant physical examination (NIPE) should be suitably trained and competent before completing any clinical examination or procedure (National Institute for Health and Care Excellence [NICE], 2014). After considering Chapters 1–5, which examined the qualities that enhance the skills of the NIPE practitioner, such as the communication skills needed to support parents throughout this examination and in relation to health promotion, this chapter moves you on to the next point in your learning. Chapter 6 subcategorises the physical examination into sections, with contributions from guest specialist authors experienced in performing the clinical examination. Similar to any medical examination, the NIPE requires preparation; in Chapter 5 you were directed how to study the mother's maternal notes to highlight and explore any areas of care that might require further examination or referral such as a family history or mode of delivery, or condition at birth so it would be good to refer back to previous chapters to support the step-by-step approach to the examination.

Before starting the examination you need to be assured that you have appropriate time allocated and are suitably free to finish the entire examination. Even for an experienced NIPE practitioner, problems can occur if the NIPE is not completed in one episode of care. Chapter 9 examines the governance and accountability related to the extended role of the NIPE practitioner, with the chapter stressing that human healthcare errors are increased when a skill or procedure is rushed (McDowell et al., 2009). Before starting the NIPE you should have discussed the NIPE process with the parents so that they are fully informed about the manner in which the examination will take place. Most trusts use a data monitoring system such as NIPE SMART, so you will require access to this system to document completion and make the relevant referrals. Before commencing the examination, ensure that you understand the monitoring system in place within your organisation and have suitable access (see Chapter 9 where an explanation of why data monitoring related to the NIPE is important to meet national standards is provided).

The NIPE is completed in all areas where mothers and babies are cared for, which can include the community setting or the neonatal unit. It is therefore important to consider the environment and ensure that there is privacy, so the parents can openly divulge any family history, and that you can explain any findings in detail. A central component to a smooth examination is ensuring that you have prepared and have access to all the equipment needed to complete the NIPE such as:

- An ophthalmoscope
- A stethoscope
- A tape measure
- A saturation monitor
- A light source to view inside the mouth
- A tongue depressor.

All the equipment needed for the NIPE is explained in greater depth during the subchapters related to the examination, in which the specialist authors break down the examination to help with your learning.

What is included in the examination has been stipulated by NICE (2014), as listed in the text box.

The physical examination should include checking the infant's:

- Appearance including colour, breathing, behaviour, activity and posture
- Head (including fontanelles), face, nose, mouth, including palate, ears, neck, and general symmetry of head and facial features. Measure and plot head circumference
- Eyes: check opacities and red reflex
- Neck and clavicles, limbs, hands, feet and digits; assess proportions and symmetry
- Heart: check position, heart rate, rhythm and sounds, murmurs and femoral pulse volume
- Lungs: check effort, rate and lung sounds
- Abdomen: check shape and palpate to identify any organomegaly; also check condition of umbilical cord
- Genitalia and anus: check for completeness and patency and undescended testes in males
- Spine: inspect and palpate bony structures and check integrity of the skin
- Skin: note colour and texture, as well as any birthmarks or rashes
- Central nervous system: observe tone, behaviour, movements and posture. Elicit newborn reflexes only if concerned
- Hips: check symmetry of the limbs and skinfolds (perform Barlow's and Ortolani's manoeuvres)
- Cry: note sound
- Weight: measure and plot

The way in which you perform the examination is not strictly set as long as you complete all the aspects stipulated by NICE. Some practitioners examine and listen to the heart and respiratory system first, if the infant is settled; this often makes this part of the examination easier because it can be challenging to hear the heart sounds if the infant is distressed and crying. It can be useful when first embarking on the experience of performing the NIPE to keep a checklist or notebook to hand. This will not only ensure that you do not miss any area of the examination but also give you the tools to keep note of the measurements and saturation monitoring levels. This information must be added to the NIPE SMART or data monitoring system on completion of the examination. This section approaches the examination from the top, starting with examination of the head.

References

McDowell, S.E., Ferner, H.S. and Ferner, R. (2009). The pathophysiology of medication errors: How and where they arise. *British Journal of Clinical Pharmacology*, **67**: 605–13.

National Institute for Health and Care Excellence (NICE) (2014). *Postnatal Care. NICE Clinical Guideline 37*. London: NICE.

6A Examination of the head, including the ears, neck, eyes and neurological (tone)

Melanie Carpenter and Michelle Scott

Introduction

A cephalocaudal approach is usually advocated for the newborn examination. Following a cephalocaudal approach means examining the head and its structures, systems and organs first. The head, neck and face of the infant will need a visual inspection, measurements obtained, palpation and the use of an ophthalmoscope for the eyes. If there are any concerns, referral should be made to a senior member of the neonatal team.

One of the four main components of NIPE screening is to assess and identify any problems with the eyes and refer for specialist assessment (Public Health England, 2018). It is estimated that around 2 or 3 in 10,000 babies will have an anomaly of the eyes, such as congenital cataracts, that requires treatment ((Public Health England, 2018). Furthermore, it is thought that another 1 in 10,000 go undiagnosed (Russell et al., 2011). Early identification and referral are essential for the treatment to be most effective.

CLINICAL TIP

Although a cephalocaudal approach is recommended for a thorough systematic approach, if the infant is quiet or sleeping at the start of the examination, it is advisable to undertake cardiac assessment first, as well as an observation of the infant's state at rest, before the physical examination.

History taking

A full and comprehensive history that incorporates family, antenatal, perinatal and postnatal history is implicit to the newborn examination. Thorough history taking helps the consultation by identifying potential risks and subsequent decision-making (Public Health England, 2018).

Important considerations before performing an examination of the head, face, neck and tone are summarised in Table 6A.1.

Examination of the head, ears, neck and eyes necessitates some understanding of neurological development, anatomy, physiology, minor and major injuries, and eye development, and includes the skull, face, mouth, palate, nose, mandible and neck.

The face starts to develop from 5 weeks' gestation. Facial clefts close. Formation of the palate and nose occurs between = weeks 6 and 9 of embryonic development. The skull forms from 4 weeks and reaches full size at around the age of 1 year, but does not completely fuse until adulthood (Sadler, 2014). The skull is made up of two easily identifiable parts, the viscerocranium, which forms the face, and the neurocranium, which forms the vault protecting the brain.

The skull

The NIPE practitioner will carefully examine the skull structures and identify red flags for congenital malformations while recognising normal variations.

Table 6A.1 History taking

Family history	Antenatal	Perinatal	Postnatal
Ethnicity	Previous antenatal history	Gestation	Midwifery or
Congenital	Single or multiple	Presentation	maternal
abnormalities	pregnancy	Type of delivery	concerns
Syndromes	Alcohol, smoking or drugs	Condition at birth	Occipitofrontal
Hearing loss	during pregnancy?	Use of scalp	circumference
Retinoblastoma	Scan findings –	electrodes	at birth
Cataracts	abnormalities.	Any documentation	Birth weight
	Growth	of vaginal lesions	Feeding
	Maternal exposure to	during delivery	
	infections and viruses		
	during pregnancy		
	including rubella,		
	toxoplasmosis, herpes		
	simplex and		
	cytomegalovirus		
	Complications during		
	pregnancy		

Assessment

The occipitofrontal circumference (OFC) should be measured using a non-stretchable paper tape measure. It is recommended that three measurements are taken and the largest of the three recorded (Baston and Durward, 2016). At term, normal measurement range is 32–37 cm. Immediately after birth the OFC may be misleading due to cranial moulding or oedema resulting from delivery.

Inspection

You will want to visualise the bone structure looking for normal skull shape and moulding. Trauma to the scalp may include bruises or lacerations from an instrument, or a puncture from a scalp electrode, and should be described according to location, size and appearance.

Palpation

Place your hands on the baby's head, feeling for the sutures using your finger-tips. Mobility of the sutures is assessed by gently placing your thumbs on either side of the suture. The anterior fontanelle should feel soft. While palpating the skull, the examiner should assess for evidence of trauma to the head, and look for the presence or absence of hair (Tappero and Honeyfield, 2016).

Fontanelles, sutures, shape and size

The fontanelles are the areas between bony plates that have not yet fused and provide flexibility to accommodate rapid brain growth during infancy. The anterior fontanelle is diamond in shape, sitting between the frontal bone and the parietal bones. It is usually between 1 cm and 5 cm and may be described as flat and soft, but should not be sunken. Bulging can occur when the infant is crying or may indicate increased intracranial pressure. It can take up to the second year before the anterior fontanelle closes. The posterior fontanelle sits between the occipital bone and the two parietal bones; it is triangular in shape, typically less than 1 cm and normally closes within 6–12 weeks (Lomax, 2015).

Sutures are the fibrous joints between two bony plates; they can be palpable at birth and their details summarised in Table A6.2 and Figure 6A.1. Sutures are approximated and mobile, and may be split by up to 1 cm. More widely spaced sutures may indicate intracranial pressure and will require further investigation (Tappero and Honeyfield, 2016).

Conditions affecting the skull

Craniosynostosis

Craniosynostosis is a rare condition defined as the premature fusion of sutures. Premature closure of the sutures will stop bone growth perpendicular to the

Table 6A.2 Summary of sutures and anatomical location

Metopic suture	Extends midline down the forehead between the two frontal bones
Coronal suture	Separates the frontal and parietal bones
Saggital suture	Extends midline from the anterior fontanelle between the two parietal bones
Lambdoidal suture	Extends posterolaterally separating the occipital from the parietal bones

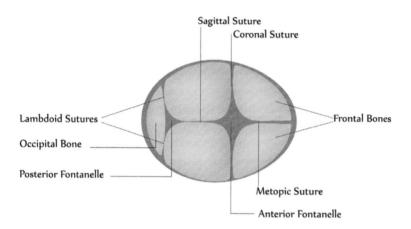

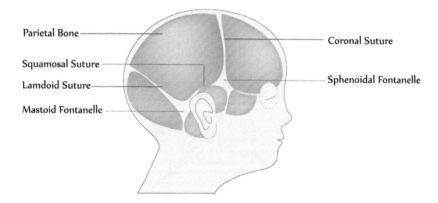

Figure 6A.1
Sutures, fontanelles and bones of the newborn cranium

suture, but will allow continued growth at the functional sutures, leading to an abnormal head shape. It may be evident at birth or become apparent later in infancy. Craniosynostosis should be suspected when there is evidence of an immobile ridge or an abnormally shaped skull. It is important to differentiate from an overriding suture (common along lambdoidal and coronal sutures), in which the bony edges overlap but are mobile and will settle. Craniosynostosis may be an isolated condition or associated with a syndrome or metabolic disorder such as hyperthyroidism (Tappero and Honeyfield, 2016). Suspected craniosynostosis will require a senior review by the medical team and referral to craniofacial specialists.

Figure 6A.2 illustrates how craniosynostosis affects head shape.

- Plagiocephaly: asymmetrical flattening of the side of the head, possibly as a result of lying in one position. It will, in the main, resolve spontaneously and does not require any action.
- Oxycephaly (turricephaly): conical or pointed appearance due to premature closing of coronal or lambdoidal sutures. This can be associated with syndromes and will need to be referred for further treatment and investigation.
- Brachycephaly: posterior flattening of the head shortening the anteroposterior diameter, which causes it to be wider than normal and sometimes can result in an enlarged forehead. Causes may include the baby be nursed on their back for long periods with little movement, intrauterine restrictions or normal moulding during delivery, or it can be indicative of some syndromes, e.g. trisomy 21.

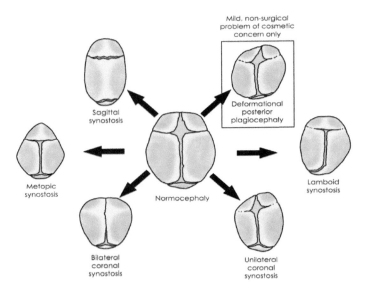

Figure 6A.2
Abnormal infant skull shapes

Caput succedaneum

Caput succedaneum is oedema secondary to prolonged pressure on the pre-senting part of the head during delivery. It can be further accentuated by a vacuum-assisted delivery. The oedema may cross the suture lines, have a poorly defined edge and be accompanied by petechiae or bruising. Caput is evident at birth and resolves spontaneously within a few days.

Cephalhaematoma

Cephalhaematoma is a collection of blood between the periosteum and the skull (Figure 6A.3). A cephalhaematoma has clearly demarcated edges confined within the suture lines; it can be bilateral or unilateral and may not be evident at birth. The most common locations are the parietal and occipital bones (Tappero and Honeyfield, 2016). Parents can be reassured that it will usually resolve within a few weeks and should be made aware that it is likely to con-tribute to jaundice.

Subgaleal haemorrhage

Subgaleal (or subaponeurotic) haemorrhage is bleeding into the space between the periosteum and the galea aponeutica of the scalp, which extends from the orbital ridges to the nape of the neck and the ears (Figure 6A.3). The risk of a subgaleal haemorrhage increases with an instrumental delivery, particularly vacuum extraction, but it can also follow a non-traumatic caesarean section or normal vaginal delivery.

Most cases of subgaleal haemorrhage are an infrequent complication of birth. It is bleeding in the large potential space between the periosteum and

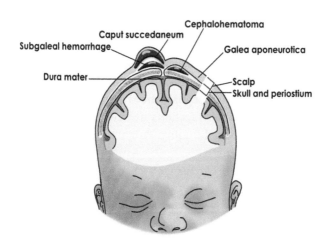

Figure 6A.3
Summary of caput, cephalhaematoma and subgaleal haemorrhage

the scalp galea aponeurosis. Clinically this will appear as a boggy mass developing over the scalp, especially over the occiput; the mass will often have superficial bruising. The swelling will develop gradually over 12–72 hours. The haematoma will spread across the calvarias; its growth is insidious and may not be recognised for a number of hours. Babies may develop dark circles around the eyes; this is known as racoon eyes. The circulating volume can be lost in this space causing haemorrhagic shock. The swelling may obscure the fontanelle and cross suture lines, distinguishing it from cephalhaematoma; on examination it is important to differentiate it from caput succedaneum and, as this can be a life-threatening condition, it should be referred immediately to the neonatal team (Gibbs et al., 2008).

An infant presenting with a generalised, rapidly growing, scalp swelling that spreads across the suture lines will require urgent referral to the neonatal team.

Cutis aplasia

Cutis aplasia is an uncommon scalp lesion that may be mistaken for a scalp wound. It is characterised by the absence of hair and skin, with or without the absence of underlying structures such as bone. Although most babies with cutis aplasia have no other abnormalities, some will have other congenital malformations.

Macrocephaly

Macrocephaly is defined as an OFC measuring above the 90th percentile for gestation on a growth chart. In some cases macrocephaly might be familial; however, there are other causes that will need to be considered and ruled out such as subgaleal haemorrhage and hydrocephalus. If the sutures are broadly spaced, an ultrasound scan should be considered.

Microcephaly

Microcephaly is an OFC of less than the 10th percentile for gestation when plotted on a growth chart. There are a number of potential aetiologies that require immediate action. Microcephaly may be due to a chromosomal or metabolic abnormality, congenital infections or antenatal exposure to alcohol or toxins. It can also be an isolated finding. Prognosis will vary depending on the extent and underlying cause.

The face

The face will provide an indication of any dysmorphic features that may be related to a syndrome. The location and relationship of the eyes, ears, nose and mouth should be assessed and noted. The forehead will normally make up a third of the face. Observe for symmetry, shape, evidence of trauma and dysmorphic features.

Facial palsy

During the NIPE, facial movements when crying are assessed. Damage to the facial nerve can result in paralysis or drooping of the affected side of the face. This condition is caused by nerve damage from application of forceps or by compression of the facial nerve during birth. It affects the overall symmetry of the face and may be accompanied by absence of forehead wrinkling, nasal labial folds and partial closing of the eye on the affected side. If the eyes cannot close fully an ophthalmological opinion should be sought. A prescription for supplemental teardrops may be required to prevent drying of the cornea and further damage to the eye. A facial palsy should show signs of improvement within 48 hours of birth, though full resolution may take several weeks. Continued facial asymmetry may be an indication of a central abnormality (Tappero and Honeyfield, 2016).

Salmon patch naevus

This is a common faint pink vascular birthmark usually seen on eyelids, the glabella (area above the nose between the eyebrows) or the nape of the neck (Figure 6A.4). Naevi on the nape of the nape may persist whereas the others will usually disappear.

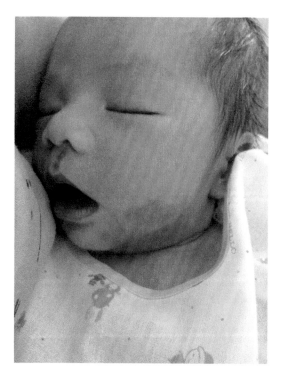

Figure 6A.4
Salmon patch naevus

The ears

The ear is a complex organ with three anatomical parts: the external (auricle), inner and middle ear. Differentiating minor defects and developmental (i.e. due to intrauterine compression) and significant defects is an important part of the examination because significant defects may be indicative of a chromosomal abnormality or syndrome.

Some ear anomalies are non-specific and there is a wide variety of insignificant structural variations that fall into the normal range.

Assessment

Assessment should include visualisation of the position, shape, size and structure of the auricle. The upper margin of the ear should be at the same level as the eyes and be similar on both sides. The external auditory meatus, also known as the ear canal, should be visualised and presence of the opening confirmed. In a term baby, the pinna will be well formed with cartilage that recoils when folded. Asymmetry of the ears may be due to the position of the infant *in utero* and is a common finding on examination. A poorly formed or unusually shaped external ear or low set ears may suggest a syndrome or chromosomal anomaly.

The normal anatomy of the ear can be seen in Figure 6A.5.

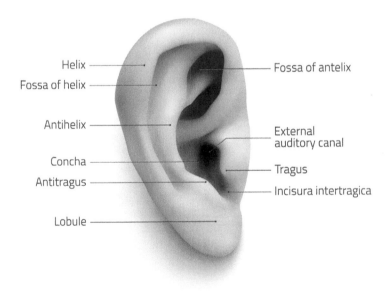

Figure 6A.5
Anatomy of outer ear and pinna

Common findings are the presence of preauricular skin tags and preauricular sinus (or pits). Skin tags are epithelial mounds that are located close to the tragus, and can be familial. Both preauricular skin tags and preauricular sinuses can be familial or associated with other abnormalities and hearing loss. A hearing test should be performed before discharge home or within the first few weeks of life, and any abnormalities followed up by a further appointment.

The eyes

Examination of the eye is principally aimed at detecting any abnormality that may interfere with visual development. It is important to have a good foundation of knowledge about the anatomy of the eye, including the shape, size, position and colour (Figure 6A.6). The distance between the outer cantha can be separated into approximately three equal segments. The sclera should be white; a blue sclera could indicate osteogenesis imperfecta and a yellow one jaundice.

Assessment

The general appearance of the eyes should be observed, including shape, position, symmetry and the newborn's ability to open them. Abnormal placement or spacing of the eyes or small palpebral fissures (openings) may suggest a syndrome or chromosomal abnormality. Swelling, bruising and oedema are

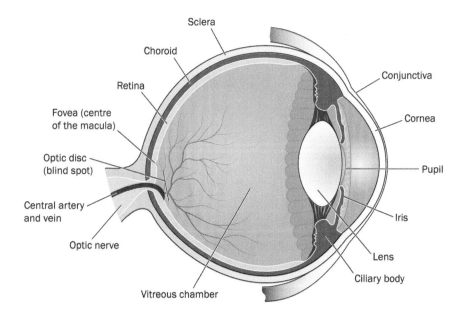

Figure 6A.6
Anatomy of the eye

common findings after a vaginal delivery. Conjunctival and subconjunctival haemorrhages are common, and occur as a consequence of the capillaries rupturing in the mucous membrane that lines the eyelids. Clinically this is seen as a bright red area in the sclera near the iris; it will usually resolve without intervention. However, the parents should be offered reassurance and, if you have any doubts, then consult a more experience practitioner for support.

Using an ophthalmoscope, at +10 dioptres (D) held approximately 15–20 cm away the examiner should direct the light at the pupils to assess for size and equality, and that they react to light (by constricting). The presence of the red reflex should be assessed. When a bright light is directed at the infant's lens, a clear red, orange or yellow colour is reflected from the retina back to the examiner. In dark-skinned infants the 'red reflex' may be paler or orange to grey in colour (Tappero and Honeyfield, 2016).

Brushfield's spots

Brushfield's spots are white or bluish spots that appear around the iris and can occasionally be seen with the naked eye. These can be a normal finding but are also associated with trisomy 21.

Epicanthic folds

Epicanthic folds describe a skinfold of the upper eyelid, which covers the inner corner of the eye. It may be a normal variant or familial, commonly seen in south-east Asian populations, but is also a typical finding in trisomy 21 (Figure 6A.7) (Lomax, 2015).

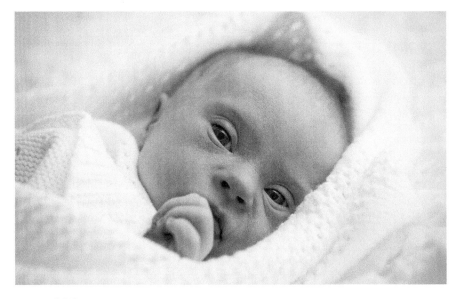

Figure 6A.7
Baby with features of trisomy 21

Blocked lacrimal ducts

Tears normally drain from the eye through small tubes called tear (lacrimal) ducts, situated between the eye and the nose. They can become blocked and the duct may fill with fluid. This normally resolves within the first few months of life and requires no treatment. Signs and symptoms may include swollen, inflamed and sometimes infected watery eyes – in particular pooling by the lacrimal punctum. Tear formation does not usually occur until the infant is aged 2–3 months and the nasolacrimal duct does not become fully patent until age 5–7 months. Eye drainage is common until the ducts are fully formed. Discharge should not be purulent and is usually watery. It may form crusting; however, it should be confirmed that it is not infective or containing pus because this might indicate a different diagnosis. Unless accompanied by signs of inflammation and redness, this can generally be treated with gentle cleansing with sterile water (Flannigan, 2011).

Eye infection

Discharge from the eye is not uncommon and the NIPE practitioner will need to differentiate between causes. Conjunctivitis and blockage of the lacrimal duct may cause discharge. Further investigation and monitoring are necessary, including obtaining eye swabs. Topical antibiotic ointment is the most effective treatment and should be considered (Tappero and Honeyfield, 2016). Prolific and persistent discharge particularly in association with erythema or swelling could be as a result of gonococcal, staphylococcal or chlamydial infections; these should be reviewed by a senior clinician for further advice.

Congenital cataracts

When lens fibres grow abnormally, the lens can vary from having small 'spots' to complete opacity of the lens. This can be hereditary, as a result of antenatal infection (e.g. rubella), or associated with a number of metabolic disorders (Table 6A.3) (Mansoor et al., 2016). Of congenital cataracts 60% result from

---

Table 6A.3 Summary of disorders associated with congenital cataracts

- Galactoseamia
- Mucolipidosis type I
- Mucolipidosis type II
- Fabry's disease
- Galactokinase deficiency
- Glucose-6-phosphate dehydrogenase deficiency
- Mannosidosis
- Refsum's disease
- Lowe's syndrome
- Alport's syndrome
- Familiar hypoparathyroidism
- Cholesterol biosynthesis defects (Smith–Lemli–Opitz syndrome, lathosterolosis)
- Metabolic syndrome
- Diabetes

---

metabolic disorders and can be associated with some syndromes, such as Cohen's syndrome, and systemic conditions, such as diabetes. Ophthalmic and genetic follow-up is necessary.

Congenital glaucoma

This is a rare condition that may be inherited. It is caused by the incorrect development of the eye drainage system before birth. This can cause raised intraocular pressure, which, left untreated, damages the optic nerve. It is most probably caused by rubella or recessive genetic mutations. It is the most common cause of macrophthalmia, a condition in which the eyeball is unusually large, or the eye is abnormally large in size due to anomalous eye development. This condition requires an urgent ophthalmic review (Mansoor et al., 2016).

Table 6A.4 gives a summary of possible abnormalities of the eye.

CLINICAL TIP

Abnormal placement of the eyes or small palpebral fissures (eye openings) can alert the examiner to the presence of a syndrome or congenital anomaly; continue the examination and alert the medical team for further advice, clearly documenting your findings.

The nose

The nose on a newborn infant will usually have a familial shape and size but is generally smaller and more flat than the nose of adults. It should be symmetrical and placed in the midline of the face. It may be squashed from the position in the uterus but this should improve within the first few weeks of life.

Babies are obligate nose breathers until a few months of age. If the nostrils are flaring, this is a sign of respiratory distress, which should be referred immediately to the medical team.

Assessment

Assess breathing while the infant is quiet, and visualise the nares. Look for position, shape, patency, work of breathing and excessive secretions/mucus and skin colour. The nose should be centrally placed and patent. Any signs of respiratory distress should prompt a senior medical review.

The tongue should fit nicely into the floor of the mouth and not be too large or protruding. Macroglossia (large tongue) is associated with the Beckwith–Wiedemann syndrome, hypothyroidism and Down's syndrome.

Table 6A.4 Summary of possible abnormalities of the eye

- Retinoblastoma: rare carcinogenic tumour, which forms on the immature cells of the retina. Can occur in one or both eyes and is likely to show up as 'white reflex' on examination. Urgent ophthalmic referral is necessary

- Aniridia: partial or complete absence of the iris, resulting in an enlarged pupil and its inability to be reactive to light. You will be expected to refer to ophthalmology

- Coloboma: a hole in one of the structures of the eye – lens, retina or iris – and is a result of early malformations in development. Can be associated with some syndromes. Genetic and ophthalmic follow-up would be standard practice in cases of coloboma

- Anophthalmia: one or both eyes are missing; this may be associated with either a syndrome or a genetic inheritance or mutation

- Microphthalmia: describes a small eye, which can be caused by congenital infections such as rubella or as a result of a syndrome. Further screening for infections and referral for ophthalmic review are necessary because vision impairment is likely

- Macrophthalmia: see also congenital glaucoma. This is a build-up of fluid, due to blocked drainage, which results in increased pressure. It can in some cases cause opacity to the cornea. This condition requires urgent ophthalmic review

- Ptosis: can occur in one or both eye and is defined by drooping of the eyelid; depending on the degree of droop, it may need referral. Is likely to be as a caused by developmental issues with the levator muscles

- Dacrocystocele: a blockage in the nasolacrimal duct, which gives rise to a bluish-grey cyst located in the inferomedial canthus

Choanal atresia or stenosis

This is a congenital defect in which the nasal passages are blocked. It can occur bilaterally or unilaterally and is more common in girls than boys. If unilateral, the infant may not show any obvious signs or symptoms. If bilateral, the infant will have difficulty breathing, especially when feeding. Referral to senior medical team or ear, nose throat department (ENT) should be made urgently, especially in cases where respiratory distress is present (in particular during feeding) because a patent airway will need to be established.

CLINICAL TIP

Infants with bilateral choanal atresia will appear cyanotic at rest and pink when crying.

The mouth

The mouth forms from the pharyngeal arches and the neural crest. The component parts include the palate, teeth and gums, tongue and lips. The palate is formed during both embryonic and fetal stages, and can lead to an isolated cleft lip, cleft lip and palate or cleft palate, depending on the extent of the developmental problem. It can be familial, as a result of chromosomal anomalies or antenatal exposure to toxins (e.g. maternal phenytoin ingestion).

Assessment

The shape and size of the oral cavity, lips, philtrum (midline groove between the nose and the upper lip) and mandible should be observed. A small oral opening is described as microstomia. A thin upper lip with a flat philtrum and short palpebral fissures (the elliptical space between the open eyelids) may be observed in fetal alcohol syndrome. An abnormally small mandible or lower jaw bone is known as micrognathia (it is vital in these babies that the palate is clearly visualised because the presence of micrognathia with cleft palate signifies the Pierre Robin sequence).

Lips and mucous membranes should be pink in colour; they may have a bluish tinge initially during the transition from intrauterine to extrauterine life, but the colour should improve within the first few hours of life. If the mucous membranes remain blue, it is important to check the baby's oxygen saturations and refer the infant to the neonatal team. The lips may be blue as a result of peripheral cyanosis (acrocyanosis), though, if of concern, pulse oximetry should be performed.

Using a tongue depressor and a torch, the entire mouth including the soft and hard palate, uvula, gums, mucous membranes and tongue should be carefully examined (Royal College of Paediatrics and Child Health, 2014). Visualisation is imperative to identify any clefts or malformations.

Ankyloglossia (tongue tie)

Tongue-tie is a common finding and may be noted where the frenulum on the underside of the tongue restricts movement of the tongue (Figure 6A.8). In severe cases the tongue may be fused in place. Tongue-tie may create feeding difficulties by interfering with positioning and attachment required for effective breastfeeding. In some cases, frenulotomy (surgical division of the frenulum) will be required. Guidelines relating to referral and assessment for frenulotomy will vary according to local hospital policy (Flannigan, 2011).

Neonatal teeth

If teeth are found, it is recommended that a referral be made to the orthodontic team. Removal may be necessary, particularly if the teeth are loose.

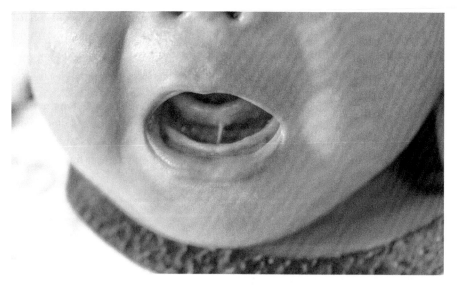

Figure 6A.8
Ankyloglossia (tongue-tie)

Cleft lip and/or palate

Around 1200 babies are born with a cleft lip and/or palate in the UK every year (RCPCH, 2014; Cleft Lip and Palate Association, 2018). A cleft lip is often detected on antenatal scan and referred to the 'cleft team'. A cleft palate will usually be diagnosed after birth.

A cleft lip (Figure 6A.9) can range from a small notch on the lip to a complete separation of the upper lip that extends into the nose. It can be unilateral or bilateral and complete (reaching the nose) or incomplete. A cleft lip may also affect the gums.

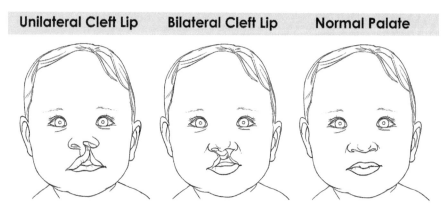

Figure 6A.9
Unilateral and bilateral cleft lip

A cleft palate is a gap in the roof of the palate. A cleft can affect the hard and soft palate. The uvula hangs from the end of the soft palate and a bifid uvula is often associated with soft palate clefts. A cleft palate may be an isolated finding, but other anomalies are often present (Flannigan, 2011; Tappero and Honeyfield, 2016).

Where possible, babies with a cleft lip and/or palate should remain with their mother. Feeding support will be required. Referral to the local cleft team after birth is vital, particularly if the family have not been seen by the cleft team antenatally. You will also need to consider genetic testing and ongoing follow-up.

Epstein's pearls

Often small white/cream clusters of spots can be seen on the junction between the hard and soft palate; these are common and known as Epstein's pearls; they disappear within the first week of life (Tappero and Honeyfield, 2016).

CLINICAL TIP

Carefully visualizing the uvula using a tongue depressor and good lighting is essential on examination.

The neck

The neck includes seven cervical vertebrae from the base of the skull to the thoracic spine. It incorporates a complex network of nerves, muscles, ligaments and major blood vessels.

THINK POINT

Consider what you might find when examining the neck.

Inspection and palpation

Visually assess the length of the neck. Does it appear shortened? To observe the neck you must visualise and palpate anteriorly, laterally and posteriorly. Elevate the shoulders to allow the head to fall back slightly; in this position the examiner should have all-round vision of the neck and observe any asymmetry, thickening or webbing. Asymmetry is often caused by intrauterine positioning, but these signs could be indicative of anomalies such as Klippel–Feil syndrome (Tappero and Honeyfield, 2016).

Klippel–Feil syndrome

This is a rare bone disorder that results in the fusion of two or more vertebrae in the neck. Associated red flag signs include: low hair line, webbed neck, torticollis, congenital scoliosis, spina bifida, respiratory problems, renal, rib and cardiac malformations, and limited movement in the neck.

Webbed neck

Webbed neck, also known as pterygium colli, is a congenital skinfold between the neck and the shoulders ,giving the webbed appearance. It is associated with syndromes such as Noonan's, Turner's and Klippel–Feil syndromes. As the NIPE practitioner presented with a baby with a webbed neck, you would be expected to assess this baby looking for other associated red flags for the above syndromes. The baby will need further observation, tests and referral for genetics and potentially surgery.

Torticollis

Torticollis is a condition when the sternocleidomastoid muscle is shorter on one side, resulting in a 'preferential' turning of the head to that side. It is thought to be the result of limited intrauterine space. Referral to physiotherapy would be advantageous even though this condition can resolve itself within 6 weeks. If left, it can result in plagiocephaly.

Pharyngeal (branchial) cleft

This congenital malformation may appear as fistulae, cysts, pits, sinuses, tags or lumps in the anterior portion of the sternocleidomastoid muscle. Due to a risk of infection you will need to refer for a surgical review.

Cystic hygroma

A cystic hygroma is the most common cyst seen in the neck and can be described as a swelling in the neck and the lymph ducts. Size can vary and may cause airway obstruction or difficulties with feeding.

Haemangioma

A haemangioma is a collection of abnormally formed blood vessels, more commonly seen on the head and neck. They form a lump under the skin and are sometimes called 'strawberry marks'. These marks are common in babies and not usually seen at birth; they develop over the following few weeks.

Superficial haemangiomas are usually a raised, bright-red area of skin. Deep haemangiomas are bluish in colour. It is important to note the position of the lump; if they are close to the eye or in the midline, they can be associated with further midline defects, an ultrasound scan or magnetic resonance imaging may be required for a full assessment.

Muscle tone

When handling the baby for NIPE, the practitioner will be undertaking an assessment of limb movement, muscle tone and reflexes (Tappero and Honeyfield, 2016).

Neurological development progresses with gestational age and this should be taken into account during the examination. Any concerns relating to tone, movement or general appearance of the baby should be escalated to the medical team because this may indicate a central nervous system, metabolic, infective or chromosomal disorder.

Assessment

Observe the baby's general appearance, position and movements while at rest and awake. After birth, a term baby will adopt a flexed position of both limbs and. hands loosely clenched. When active, limb movements should be smooth, varied and symmetrical. Lack of movement may indicate injury or nerve damage (Baston and Durward, 2016).

Muscle strength is determined by assessing posture, tone and neonatal reflexes (summarised in Table 6A.5). The examiner should also test resistance of the extremities using passive movements, and confirm arm and leg recoil.

Postural tone may be evaluated by performing a pull-to-sit manoeuvre by grasping both hands, slowly pulling the baby from the supine to the sitting position while examining the degree of head lag. The general tone may be assessed by placing the hands under each axilla and holding the baby. A baby with normal tone will remain supported and not 'slip'. When newborns are placed prone, supported in one hand, those with normal tone will attempt to raise their head and legs.

If the baby is awake and crying, observe the quality of the cry and the symmetry of movement. A weaker cry may be heard in premature infants and a high-pitched cry may be evident with neurological disturbances, metabolic abnormalities or drug withdrawal.

Hypotonia

Hypotonia refers to reduced tone or 'floppiness' and is the most common neurological abnormality observed during the NIPE; it requires medical follow-up. Hypotonia may be generalised or more apparent in either the upper or the lower limbs, or unilateral (Lomax, 2015).

Table 6A.5 Summary of reflexes to be assessed during the NIPE
• **Suck**: present at birth in response to stimulus of touching/stroking the lips. Using a gloved finger, mouth opens and sucking occurs. Strength and coordination of suck are evaluated
• **Rooting**: stroke the cheek and corner of the mouth. Infant will turn head towards the stimulus
• **Palmar grasp**: placing finger in the palm of the hand, infant will grasp the finger. Grasp should tighten when there is an attempt to withdraw finger
• **Moro's reflex**: place baby in a supine position with the infant's head in the examiner's palm. The examiner should then carefully allow the infant's neck to extend. If Moro's reflex is present, the infant will respond by extending and abducting both arms and open hands, followed by inward movement, some flexion of the arms and clenching of fists. Observe for symmetry
• **Tonic neck**: place baby in supine position and turn head to one side. The upper arm on side where the head is turned will extend and the opposite arm flexes. This is also known as the 'fencing position'
• **Stepping**: when held upright, allowing the feet to touch a flat surface, stepping movements can be observed
• **Babinski's response**: a response to stimulation of the sole of the foot. Extension or flexion of the toes should occur

(Lissauer et al., 2015)

Hypertonia

This is less common than hypotonia and refers to increased tone or 'stiffness'. Arching of the back may be seen in meningitis, severe encephalopathy or intraventricular haemorrhage. Any concerns with an infant's tone should lead to a medical review before discharge (Tappero and Honeyfield, 2016).

Jitteriness

Jitteriness is a common finding and characterised by rapid alternating movements of equal amplitude in both directions; it generally occurs in response to environmental stimuli (noise or touch). It can be stopped by flexing and holding the affected limb.

Jitteriness is distinct from the abnormal movements associated with seizures because they are stimulus sensitive, whereas seizures are not. Jitteriness has symmetrical tremors, whereas seizure may be focal; an infant with jitteriness will not have accompanying autonomic physiological changes such as apnoea, tachycardia and hypertension.

Excessive jitteriness can occur with drug withdrawal, hypoglycaemia and hypocalcaemia, so it is important to confirm antenatal history and check blood glucose level. Tests may also be performed to determine calcium and magnesium levels (Flannigan, 2011).

End of chapter quiz

1   What are the differences between caput succedaneum and cephalhaematoma?
2   Name the sutures and describe their positions on the skull.
3   What clinical findings would alert the NIPE practitioner to the possibility of a chromosomal abnormality or syndrome?
4   Why is it important to use a tongue depressor and light source when examining the mouth?
5   How would you manage a baby who appears to be 'jittery' on examination?

References

Baston, H. and Durward, H. (2016). *Examination of the Newborn*, 3rd edn. London, Routledge.

Flannigan, C. (2011). *A Practical Guide to Managing Paediatric Problems on the Postnatal Wards*. Oxford: Radcliffe Publishing.

Gibbs, R.S., Danforth, N., Karlan, B.Y. and Haney, A.F. (2008). *Danforth's Obstetric and Gynaecology*. Philadelphia, PA: Lippincott Williams & Wilkins, p. 470.

Lissauer, T., Fanaroff, A.A., Miall, L. and Fanaroff, J. (2015). *Neonatology at a Glance*, 3rd edn. Chichester: John Wiley & Sons.

Lomax, A. (2015). *Examination of the Newborn. An evidence-based guide*, 2nd edn. Chichester: John Wiley & Sons Ltd.

Mansoor, N., Mansoor, T., and Ahmed, M. (2016). Eye pathologies in neonates. *International Journal of Ophthalmology*, **9**: 1832–8.

Public Health England (2018). *Newborn and Infant Physical Examination: Programme handbook. Changes to NIPE programme standards and handbook*. London: Public Health England.

Royal College of Paediatrics and Child Health (2014). *Palate Examination: Identification of cleft palate in the newborn*. London: RCPCH.

Russell, H.C., McDougall, V.M. and Dutton, G.N. (2011). Congenital cataract. *British Medical Journal*, **342**: d3075.

Sadler, T.W. (2014). *Langman's Medical Embryology*, 13th edn, Philadelphia, PA: Wolters-Kluwer.

Tappero, E.P. and Honeyfield, M.E. (2016). *Physical Assessment of the Newborn: A comprehensive approach to the art of physical examination*. New York: Springer Publishing Co.

6B Cardiovascular examination of the newborn infant

Jonathan Hurst

Introduction

Examination of the cardiovascular system is one of the four main domains of the newborn infant physical examination (NIPE) screening programme (Public Health England, 2018), to detect congenital heart defects. Congenital heart disease is one of the most common groups of congenital abnormalities, with approximately 4–10 cases per 1000 (i.e. just under 1%) of live births (Public Health England, 2018), with around 2–3 cases per 1000 being serious or critical, requiring urgent management. Undiagnosed heart defects still remain a major cause of avoidable death in early infancy, reduced significantly by a careful, thorough examination as part of the newborn screening programme, which allows for earlier detection and intervention.

For many new NIPE practitioners, the cardiovascular examination causes the most concern, especially with the knowledge that, even with careful examination, some congenital heart conditions may not be detectable. Also, it is important for the NIPE practitioner to be able to distinguish signs consistent with the transition from intrauterine to extrauterine life, from those of significant underlying cardiac issues. Examination of the cardiovascular system extends much further than just listening for the presence of a heart murmur, which may still not be present in a significant cardiac lesion in the early newborn period. Therefore, a careful systematic approach to the examination of this system is required, which is the main aim of this chapter to highlight and explain the relevance of any signs established.

Fetal cardiac screening

The fetal heart is routinely examined at the time of the fetal anomaly ultrasound scan between 18^{+0} and 20^{+6} weeks' gestation (National Health Service Screening Programmes, 2015), to screen for major fetal anomalies. At this time, the four chambers of the heart are visualised, along with the outflow tracts from each ventricle. Despite this scan, the detection rate for serious cardiac anomalies, is around 50% (NHS Screening Programmes, 2015), with septal defects, coarctation of the aorta and abnormal connections of the pulmonary veins being some of the common conditions missed, due to the limitations of scanning and the fact that the fetal circulation is dependent on the presence of a ductus arteriosus, a muscular artery connecting the main pulmonary arteries and the aorta (the outflow tracts), which may disguise problems with narrowing of or blockages in these vessels. Since 2016, additional views of the fetal upper mediastinum (three-vessel and trachea view [3VT]) have been added to the standard views taken, although this has not yet been evaluated in terms of the impact on the detection rates of congenital heart disease (NHS Screening Programmes, 2015).

Fetal echocardiography is generally reserved for 'high-risk' pregnancies, those where there is a significant family history of structural heart disease, other abnormalities seen on fetal scanning that may be associated with a cardiac lesion, or certain maternal health diseases that are associated with an increased risk of fetal cardiac problems (e.g. diabetes). This can be performed from 13 weeks' gestation, i.e. after the first trimester dating scan, when the fetal nuchal fold is looked at. Even fetal echocardiography only has an 85% detection rate for congenital heart problems.

CLINICAL TIP

If there are cardiac abnormalities suspected from the antenatal scan, this warrants a senior paediatric review. However, normal antenatal scans do not rule out significant congenital cardiac defects.

Cardiac lesions in the newborn

As mentioned, congenital heart disease affects approximately 4–10 per 1000 live births, with around a third being symptomatic in the newborn period. By far the most common are ventricular septal defects (VSDs), followed by atrial septal defects (ASDs) and patent ductus arteriosus (PDA) (Hoffmann and Kaplan, 2002). Cyanotic congenital heart lesions, such as transposition of the great arteries (TGA), tricuspid atresia or right ventricular outflow tract obstruction (pulmonary atresia or critical stenosis), are collectively rarer, although they can be life threatening, if not detected early after birth. Coarctation of the aorta and other left ventricular outflow tract obstructions (critical aortic stenosis, hypoplastic left heart, interrupted aortic arch) tend to present with collapse if not found early, especially when the ductus arteriosus, which provides a method of blood bypassing the defect, closes in the first few days of life. Again these are rare, although they have highly significant consequences if not picked up in the early newborn period. Unfortunately, these lesions are not always found antenatally, hence the need for a structured newborn assessment of the cardiovascular system being vital.

It is well known that infants with a chromosomal abnormality have a higher risk of associated congenital heart disease. Down's syndrome, otherwise known as trisomy 21, one of the most common chromosomal abnormalities, can be associated with a range of different congenital heart lesions in around 40% of cases (atrioventricular septal defects [AVSDs], VSDs and ASDs in isolation, tetralogy of Fallot). Any infant found to have a chromosomal abnormality should have an echocardiogram as part of their care pathway to assess for the presence of congenital heart disease. The converse is also true, in that detection of a cardiac lesion may be the presentation of an underlying genetic issue (or part of a constellation of features, such as in 22q11 deletion (previously known as DiGeorge's syndrome or CATCH-22), or in the VACTERL association (vertebral, anorectal, cardiac, tracheo-oesophageal, renal and limb abnormalities).

CLINICAL TIP

Any infant with dysmorphic features warrants a senior paediatric review and consideration for an early echocardiogram.

Cardiovascular adaptation at birth

As a NIPE practitioner, it is important that you understand the changes that are happening in the transitional period from intrauterine to extrauterine life. It is around this time that you will be performing the initial NIPE, and hence you may find signs relating to this transition, as you may do in the vast majority of term or near term infants. You may also pick up that the transition is not occurring as it should, and need to refer on for an urgent senior paediatric assessment. Hence, it is useful to understand how the two circulations differ, and the changes that need to happen. These changes do not all happen at the same time, which is one of the reasons why some cardiac defects cannot be picked up on the initial examination in the immediate newborn period.

THINK POINT

Why is it important for a NIPE practitioner to have an understanding of the changes that are taking place in the transitional period from intrauterine to extrauterine life?

Fetal (intrauterine) circulation

Oxygenated and nutrient-rich blood flows from the placenta to the fetal liver via the umbilical vein. Approximately 80% flows through the liver (portal system), whereas the other 20% bypasses the liver through the ductus venosus. Both systems then enter the inferior vena cava, and into the right atrium of the heart.

Most of the blood entering the right atrium then passes over to the left atrium via the foramen ovale. This blood enters the left ventricle and then the aorta, which supplies the fetal organs, and then returns to the placenta via the two umbilical arteries (now deoxygenated).

A small amount of blood that enters the right atrium, mainly from the superior vena cava (the large vein draining blood from the fetal head and neck veins back to the heart), then flows into the right ventricle and onwards into the pulmonary artery.

The fetal lungs are filled with fluid, which leads to the pulmonary vessels to the lungs being constricted, creating a high resistance to any blood flow from the heart to the lungs. So only a very small amount of blood then flows on to the lungs (enough for them to grow), which in turn comes back to the left atrium via the pulmonary veins. In fact, the blood flow to the fetal lung is about an eighth of that going to the newborn lung (if the infant undergoes the transition correctly). There is no need for the fetal lungs to allow significant amounts of gas exchange, due to the presence of the placenta.

The remainder of the blood in the main fetal pulmonary artery bypasses the lungs, due to high pressures in the pulmonary vessels via the wide-open ductus arteriosus, connecting the main pulmonary artery and the aorta, which then, as mentioned above, supplies the fetal organs and returns to the placenta via the two umbilical arteries.

Neonatal (extrauterine) circulation

As the newborn infant takes its first breaths, or if effective positive pressure breaths are administered to the infant, the lungs (specifically alveoli) inflate with air, displacing the fluid, which subsequently causes the pulmonary vessels around the alveoli to dilate, and the pulmonary vascular resistance to start to drop. This then causes an eightfold increase in the amount of the blood going to the lungs from the main pulmonary artery and becoming oxygenated, which returns back to the left atrium of the heart, via the pulmonary veins.

As this is taking place, the placenta has been clamped and cut, leading to a large reduction in the amount of blood now coming into the inferior vena cava and consequently the right atrium. This, coupled with the reduction in the pulmonary vascular resistance, causes the pressures in the right side of the heart to begin to fall. As more blood returns from the lungs into the left atrium, the left atrial pressures starts to rise, eventually becoming higher than that of the right atrium, causing the flap-like foramen ovale to start to close.

The umbilical vein tends to collapse and close, turning into a ligament (ligamentum teres) in the first 2 weeks of life, especially when the ductus venosus closes after 1 week (becoming the ligamentum venosum) (Avery et al., 2005). The foramen ovale does not completely shut for several months (Blackburn, 2007), and in some people may remain open (known as a patent foramen ovale or PFO). However, if the pulmonary blood flow is established as mentioned above, any flow across this flap tends to be from the higher pressure left atrium to the lower pressure right atrium. If the pulmonary circulation is not established, the right-to-left flow can remain, with the infant presenting as cyanosed.

The final 'fetal' structure to close is the ductus arteriosus. The increasing pulmonary blood flow leads to a rise in the arterial oxygen concentration in the aorta and ductus arteriosus. This triggers the smooth muscle in the wall of the ductus to contract, and subsequently the blood flow across the duct to stop. Also, the prostaglandins present around the time of labour then become metabolised and no longer have such an effect on keeping the ductus open (Askin, 2009). However, the ductus arteriosus does not always close straight away, even in healthy term newborn infants. This process can take up to 72–96 hours (3–4 days) for the blood flow to stop across the ductus, and several weeks before it physically closes, becoming the ligamentum arteriosus. In the first few days, if the infant is transitioning normally, the pressure in the aorta will be higher than that in the pulmonary artery and there can still be flow from the aorta (left outflow tract) to the pulmonary artery (right outflow tract) (i.e. left to right). As the duct closes, there is a higher pressure of blood flowing across the duct, and hence a murmur can be heard. While the infant is transitioning, or if the infant has not established good respiratory effort, and the pulmonary vascular resistance remains high for some reason, there can be shunting of blood 'right to left' across this duct, and the infant may appear cyanosed.

It is important for the NIPE practitioner to be aware that certain congenital heart defects may not present until the transition to extrauterine life is complete, for example coarctation of the aorta may not be *fully* apparent until the ductus arteriosus has closed (though in some cases there are clinical findings, such as reduced volume femoral pulses), and large VSDs tend not to present until the pulmonary vascular resistance has fallen, which can take 2–4 weeks (see later). However, the presence of any murmur or positive sign on cardiovascular examination should be taken seriously and investigated early in the neonatal period (Kenner and Wright Lott, 2007), involving a review by a senior paediatrician – the urgency of such a review will depend on the suspected condition, though commonly it should involve a review within 24 hours of a positive finding (Public Health England, 2018) and before discharge of the infant.

> **THINK POINT**
>
> Significant cardiac defects may not be obvious at the initial NIPE in the newborn period. Consider what specific information needs to be given to parents as to what to look out for and how to seek urgent attention if any concerns arise.

History taking (associated risk factors)

It is customary to review the maternal notes and establish whether there are particular risk factors or parental concerns before performing the examination; for the purposes of detecting congenital heart disease or its risk factors, this would need further review by an experienced paediatrician if present. The following points are pertinent for any NIPE practitioner to establish (Public Health England, 2018):

- Family history of congenital heart disease (first-degree relative): this may include prior history of children with heart disease requiring significant medical or surgical intervention
- Fetal trisomy 21 (or other trisomy detected): who have a high risk of cardiac defects (see above)
- Cardiac abnormality on an antenatal scan.

The following risk factors are associated with congenital heart disease and would require, at the very least, discussion with a paediatrician, for further review (Public Health England, 2018):

- Maternal exposure to viruses, particularly in the first trimester, e.g. rubella
- Maternal systemic health issues, e.g. type 1 diabetes, epilepsy, systemic lupus erythematosus (SLE)
- Maternal teratogenic medications, e.g. antiepileptics, antipsychotic/psychotropic drugs.

Clinical symptoms about which the parents or staff caring for the infant should be asked include:

- Any breathlessness or colour change at rest or when feeding
- Any difficulty with feeding, such as whether the infant appeared tired, lethargic, quiet, reluctant to feed – or any change to feeding patterns.

CLINICAL TIP

If any of the above symptoms are present, a close examination is warranted; this could be the first presentation of significant congenital heart disease. If parents notice these, this warrants urgent review.

Examination

General

The ideal environment for the cardiovascular examination is in a well-lit and quiet room, with the infant in a calm state. As a NIPE practitioner, you will know this to be a luxury that is rarely the case, so you will have to be opportunistic with your examination, for example feeling pulses and auscultating the heart. However, if you do alter your examination routine, it is still vital to return to complete the rest of the examination of the cardiovascular system later.

Before handling the infant, you will be able to observe much about the cardiovascular status of the infant. First, does the infant look normal, or similar to the parents, if present? Are there any unusual or dysmorphic features (for example, epicanthic folds and flattened nasal bridge present in infants with trisomy 21 or Down's syndrome)? The presence of dysmorphic features raises the likelihood of an underlying associated cardiac lesion, and any infant with a chromosomal abnormality should have a formal echocardiogram. Any infant with unusual features should be reviewed by a senior paediatrician before discharge or within 24 hours of its detection.

CLINICAL TIP

Be opportunistic! Listen for heart sounds, extra sounds and murmurs while the infant is quiet. Remember, so many clues can be obtained before even auscultating the chest and heart.

What is the overall colour and perfusion of the infant? These features can be difficult to fully appreciate in the first couple of hours after birth, and also depending on the environment in which the examination is performed. If in doubt, it is important to perform pulse oximetry, both pre-ductal (right arm/wrist/hand) and post-ductal (legs) (see later for more information). Also, it is important to note, for male NIPE practitioners, that colour blindness can affect a practitioner's ability to detect mild cyanosis, and cyanosis is usually apparent only when the oxygen saturations are around 80% (Rennie, 2012). To look for true central cyanosis, it is vital to look at the mucous membranes and tongue.

However, the visual detection of central cyanosis can be subjective among healthcare professionals. If present, or any suspicion of central cyanosis is present, it needs confirming with pulse oximetry and investigating further immediately. Peripheral cyanosis (acrocyanosis) is a commonly found sign, a normal feature of the early postnatal transition, usually found as blue discoloration of the hands/feet/outer lips due to circulatory instability in the first 24–48 hours of age.

It is important, ideally while the infant is at rest, to count the respiratory rate, and observe the size/shape of the chest and any increased work of breathing (grunting noises, retraction of the intercostal muscles or abnormal breathing pattern using the abdominal muscles). Normally, the respiration rate should be around 30–40 breaths/minute, with a small amount of variation. Tachypnoea (high respiratory rate), especially above 60 breaths/min, is one of the first signs of an unwell infant, and warrants further investigation, whether or not there were coinciding signs of increased work of breathing.

Pulses and perfusion

The pulses cause much angst to the NIPE practitioner, although can be difficult to feel if the infant is very active. You may have to be opportunistic as to when you palpate them, but never miss them out. In the infant, the best, and easiest, pulses to feel are the brachial and femoral (Figure 6B.1). The brachial pulse is palpable in the medial (or inside) edge of the antecubital fossa. The femoral pulse is palpable midway between the end of the hip bone and the pubic symphysis (middle of the pubic bone), beneath the skin crease in the groin. One of the common issues for not feeling these is that the practitioner pushes too hard and obliterates the pulse completely. This pulse usually has a rate around 120–160 beats/min (much faster than even the nervous NIPE practitioner!). It is vital to palpate the pulses for their rate (counted over 15 seconds) and volume/strength.

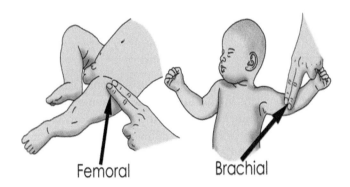

Femoral   Brachial

Figure 6B.1
Brachial and femoral pulses

Weak femoral pulses, or femoral pulses not in sync with the brachial pulses, especially if the latter are easy to feel, could be a sign of a coarctation (narrowing) of the aorta or poor perfusion, and would warrant an urgent review by a senior paediatrician or senior neonatal practitioner. A 'bounding' (very easy to feel) femoral pulse could indicate that the ductus arteriosus is still patent. If either of the pulses has an irregular rhythm, then it would be wise to have the infant reviewed and an electrocardiogram (ECG) undertaken.

CLINICAL TIP

If you cannot palpate or have difficulty palpating the femoral pulses, ask a colleague; if still unsure, arrange for an urgent senior paediatric review.

To make a crude assessment of the infant's perfusion, the capillary refill time should be established. This is done by applying gentle pressure to the sternum with the practitioner's index finger for 5 seconds, then releasing it and counting the number of seconds it takes for the skin to pink up again. The normal response is less than 2 seconds. A delay in this is a sign of poor blood flow to the skin, and can be a sign of poor perfusion, although it is also seen when the infant is cold. If abnormal, a low temperature needs to be excluded and a review arranged, especially if there are any other signs of the infant being unwell.

Examination of the heart

Before reaching for your stethoscope, it is important to establish the position of the heart (Figure 6B.2), and especially the apex (the strongest beat and most accurate place to listen for the heart rate). The presence of any heaves or thrills, though rare in the newborn examination, may indicate that the heart muscle is working harder than usual or there is a problem with the heart valves. The NIPE practitioner should place their hand gently across the sternum and chest, with fingers stretched out into the axilla. The point where you feel the heart beat most strongly is the *apex*, the area where you will hear or feel if there are problems with the mitral valve. This is usually situated in the *left* fourth intercostal space (Rennie, 2012), in the mid-clavicular line (approximately around the left nipple).

If the apex is found further round into the axilla, this is a sign that the left ventricle could be dilated and under strain. If you feel a large impulse, or *heave*, under the palm of your hand, when feeling for the apex, it could be a sign that the right ventricle could be dilated and under strain. If you cannot feel the apex beat on the left side, just check the opposite side of the chest, in case the infant has dextrocardia – this occurs in around 1 in 12,000 births (Bohun et al., 2007).

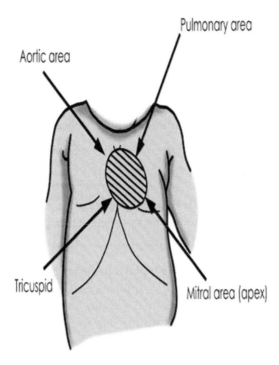

Figure 6B.2
Position of the heart

After locating the apex beat, it is useful to place the flat of your index and middle fingers over the different valve areas, to feel for any 'rumbling' sensation, akin to a cat purring, called a *thrill*, which may be suggestive of a loud murmur at the valve. These areas are:

- Apex – mitral valve
- Lower left sternal border, fourth intercostal space – tricuspid valve
- Upper left sternal border, second intercostal space – pulmonary valve
- Upper right sternal border, second intercostal space – aortic valve.

It is these areas that you are going to come back to with your stethoscope and examine further.

Heart sounds and murmurs

Many NIPE practitioners feel very uneasy and nervous when it comes to detecting murmurs and also timing the murmur, discussing its quality or locating its loudest position and where it radiates to. However, it is at this point that a knowledge of the transitional circulation and a thorough history and examination of the cardiovascular system, as outlined above, may give you some clues as to whether or not you are expecting to hear a murmur. By being methodical and trying to concentrate on specific parts of the heart sounds, it becomes easier to establish what it happening. By having a logical approach to your examination, it is less likely that significant abnormalities will be missed (Bedford and Lomax, 2015). Also, it is wise to use a fully functioning stethoscope in good condition, with no breaks in the tubing/ear pieces/diaphragm. Out of the three head sizes that are on the market, the *paediatric* size is usually the most beneficial for examining the newborn (with an adult-sized stethoscope head, one may hear heart, breath and bowel sounds all at once!) The neonatal size should be reserved for the most premature infants. Usually the murmurs are of low frequency (compared with breath sounds) and the bell (domed part) is best for hearing these. It is good practice to examine all areas with both the diaphragm and the bell.

When auscultating the heart, there are three main aspects to concentrate on:

1   Rate and rhythm
2   Heart sounds
3   Abnormal sounds/murmurs.

We have already briefly discussed 'rate and rhythm' in relation to pulses, although the most accurate way of assessing this is by auscultation of the apex. As already mentioned, the normal rate is around 120–160 beats/min. To assess this it may be wise to listen for 15 seconds and then multiply your findings by 4 (another method would be to listen for 6 seconds and then multiply by 10, though you would only be gaining a brief snapshot of the overall rate). If the infant is agitated, it is not uncommon for the heart rate to rise dramatically, sometimes even above 200 beats/min, although this should decrease as the infant settles. Persistent tachycardia warrants a senior paediatrician review and consideration given to performing an ECG. As well as the rate, the NIPE practitioner should assess for the rhythm, or regularity, of the heartbeats. It is not uncommon to find brief slowing of the heart rate as the infant breathes in, and quickening on breathing out; this is known as sinus arrhythmia, and is fully benign and requires no further follow-up. Occasional ectopic beats are also not uncommon, although if frequent or there is any concern over the nature of these beats, a senior paediatrician review and ECG should be sought.

Next, you should concentrate on listening to the heart sounds, by starting in the apex, then moving around to the left sternal edge (tricuspid area) and both the pulmonary and aortic areas.

There should be two distinct heart sounds. This first heart sound, sounding 'lub', is due to the closure of the tricuspid and mitral valves (atrioventricular valves) (Figure 6B.3). This is usually loudest at the apex, as the mitral valve makes up most of the intensity of this sound. After this, the ventricles then contract, from the apex upwards, pushes blood up into the aorta and pulmonary arteries. This period, between the first and second heart sounds is known as (ventricular) *systole*. At the end of this period, the arterial walls recoil and the pulmonary and aortic valves (semilunar valves) close, which produces the

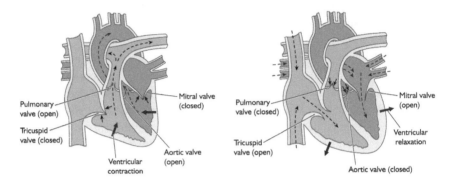

Figure 6B.3
Closure of heart valves. The first heart tone (S1), is caused by the closure of the mitral and tricuspid valves at the beginning of ventricular contraction (systole). The second heart tone (S2), is caused by the closure of the aortic and pulmonary valves at the end of the ventricular systole.

second heart sound, sounding 'dub'. The second heart sound is usually heard loudest in the upper left sternal edge. Occasionally two parts to the second heart sound may be heard, sounding 'du-dub'. The gap between the pulmonary and aortic valves closing is tiny (around 0.02–0.03 second, though this can increase slightly if the infant is breathing in). The ventricles then relax, entering *diastole*. If there are any other heart sounds heard, this could be due to an issue with the heart valves or increased flow into the ventricles. This is rare and a senior paediatric opinion should be sought.

Having established the heart sounds, you have now established 'systole' and 'diastole' (relating to the contraction and relaxation of the ventricles, respectively). A murmur is actually an *absence* of silence between these heart sounds, so you are more likely to pick it up if you have already focused on the heart sounds themselves. One of the most common pitfalls is confusing the infant's breathing for a murmur.

CLINICAL TIP

A murmur is an absence of silence between the heart sounds. Focus on the heart sounds first, then listen for any noise in between these. Keep listening and look at the infant's chest – a murmur should be persistent (also, if the infant is really breathing at 120–160 breaths/min, then this needs an urgent review anyway!).

As a NIPE practitioner you will find that you have to be opportunistic when listening to murmurs.

When listening to murmurs it is important to comment on their intensity/ loudness, timing (systolic/diastolic – see later), place where it is heard loudest, and whether the sound radiates. Examples below should make sense of this. Regarding intensity, murmurs are usually given a grade, depending on how easy it is to hear them:

- Grade 1: very soft, just about audible, (historically heard usually only by experts/those with excellent hearing abilities)
- Grade 2: soft though comfortably audible
- Grade 3: loud, easily heard by stethoscope
- Grade 4: loud, with a thrill palpable (see above)
- Grade 5: murmur heard with rim of stethoscope hardly on the chest
- Grade 6: murmur heard with stethoscope off the chest.

(Grade 5 and 6 murmurs, which are both extremely rare, are reserved for systolic murmurs only.)

You may hear other NIPE practitioners referring to the murmurs by their grade, hence including this here. However, the important point is whether you hear the murmur or not!

Heart murmurs fall into two main categories: innocent or abnormal. Innocent murmurs are due to blood flowing through normal, albeit small, orifices. They tend to be more prominent with increasing heart rates, very soft (grade 1 or 2), systolic, localised (usually left sternal edge) with no radiation, normal pulses and an otherwise normal examination. However, if concerned, it is always safer to have such babies reviewed.

Abnormal murmurs are due to blood flowing through an abnormal valve or hole in the heart, which creates turbulent blood flow. Blood flows from a high pressure to a lower pressure, which may give some clues as to where such a murmur may radiate. With regard to timing of a murmur, as well as describing it in relation to systole or diastole, it is important to comment on whether it is present throughout systole (pansystolic, i.e. heard all the way through systole, commonly obscuring the heart sounds – from the Greek 'παν' [pan] = all), clearly separate from the first heart sound although then increasing in intensity up to the second heart sound (ejection systolic), or present throughout systole and diastole (though usually louder in systole – usually described as 'machinery') (continuous). Other ways of describing the timing are using the words 'early' and 'late' to qualify the position heard in systole or diastole.

Examples of common murmurs, and their characteristics, are included in Table 6B.1.

Pure diastolic murmurs, as found in conditions such as aortic valve incompetence, are extremely rare in newborn infants. Any concern with this should be reviewed by a senior paediatrician within 24 hours. As well as the four valvular areas described above, it is important to auscultate underneath the left clavicle (common site for PDA) and in between the scapulae (radiation for coarctation).

Table 6B.1 Common murmurs on newborn examination

Defect	Picture	Intensity	Timing	Location (loudest)	Radiation	Notes
Ventricular septal defect (VSD)		Harsh	Pansystolic	Lower left sternal edge	Lower right sternal edge/none	Commonly not heard initially until right sided heart pressure decrease
Patent ductus arteriosus (PDA)		Machinery	Continuous (systole & diastole)	Under left clavicle	None	Most common in early period. Has a 'grumbling' quality. Peak intensity in mid systole
Pulmonary stenosis (PS)			Ejection systolic	2nd left intercostal space	To apex (top) of left lung	If severe, may hear an added 'click' after the first heart sound (opening of stenotic valve), and increased split second heart sound
Aortic stenosis (AS)			Ejection systolic	2nd right intercostal space	Neck	If severe, may hear an added 'click' after the first heart sound (opening of stenotic valve)
Coarctation of aorta (CoA)			Mid systolic	Under left clavicle	Back/mid scapula	FEEL THE FEMORALS! Depending on the site of the coarctation (preductal/ductal), the femoral pulses may be felt, until the duct closes

Extracardiac examination

It is important for the NIPE practitioner to bear in mind that cardiac disease commonly has a secondary effect on other organ systems. Auscultation of the lung bases may reveal crepitations (crackles), which may signify heart failure, although this is rarely present on newborn examination in the first few days of life due to high pulmonary pressures (and tend to present at 2–4 weeks of age). However, persistent tachypnoea or respiratory difficulty needs an urgent senior paediatrician review. Another important sensitive sign of heart failure and fluid overload, which can present earlier, is downward displacement and enlargement of the liver. Usually the edge of the liver may be palpable; in heart failure this enlarges dramatically, becoming palpable a few centimetres underneath the costal margin and warrants urgent review.

Pulse oximetry

The pulse oximeter provides an objective method for the detection of cyanosis, which can be clinically difficult. To obtain an optimal trace, the light from the saturation probe must be able to pass directly through an arterial flow. Poor peripheral perfusion and excess surrounding light can affect the oximeter reading of the pulsatile signal. In this case, especially if the tracing or 'pleth' is low, then it is vital to reapply the probe and consider shielding it from excess light with a PosiWrap or other light-shielding method. It is also important to allow time for the machine to achieve a steady reading, increasing its reliability. Attaching the probe to the infant, switching the pulse oximeter machine on, and then connecting the two together and leaving it in place for 30–60 seconds allow a steady, accurate tracing and reading to be achieved. A settled infant will result in a more stable, reliable and accurate reading.

CLINICAL TIP

Cyanosis (especially mild) can be difficult to detect, especially for some males with colour blindness. If you have any concerns about colour, ensure that you measure the oxygen saturations.

Over the last 20 years, routine use of pulse oximetry to detect respiratory and cardiac problems in the newborn infant has been suggested (Katzman, 1995). In this time, multiple large-scale international studies have been undertaken to investigate the effectiveness of pulse oximetry in detecting congenital heart disease (Richmond et al., 2002; Koppel et al., 2003; Reich et al., 2003; Riede et al., 2010), with some countries now adopting it as routine practice in examination of the newborn.

From July 2015 to December 2015, a large-scale newborn pulse oximetry pilot study was undertaken by Public Health England across 15 NHS trusts in England to evaluate the feasibility of implementing pulse oximetry as an addition to the NIPE programme. Over 32,000 babies were screened, performing pre-ductal (right hand) and post-ductal (foot) pulse oximetry in the first 24 hours of age. A positive result, requiring further investigation, was pulse oximetry of less than 95% in either limb or a difference between the pre- and post-ductal measurements of more than 2%; 239 infants had a positive screen. Of these, eight had critical congenital heart disease identified, with only two babies being missed by pulse oximetry (Public Health England, 2017).

This large-scale study, along with many other studies and economical evaluations, are still being deliberated as to whether it is feasible to include newborn pulse oximetry in the UK screening programme. A previous cost-effectiveness

CASE STUDY
CARDIAC ABNORMALITY ON NIPE

Eve was born at 38^{+5} weeks' gestation by normal vaginal delivery, weighing 3.2kg. Her mother, Helen, was a primigravida, who had had an uneventful, midwifery-led pregnancy, with a normal anomaly scan.

They were transferred to the postnatal ward, because Helen wished to stay in hospital overnight to have some support from the midwives in helping her establish breastfeeding. Eve latched on well and breastfeeding was becoming more established; at the time of her NIPE, she had passed urine and meconium. There were no concerns from the midwifery team or her mother about her general condition. There were no concerns about Helen's health during pregnancy and no family history of congenital heart disease.

On examination at the time of her NIPE (aged 16 hours of age), Eve was alert and content, though active in her cot. She had a respiratory rate of around 45–50 breaths/min, with no increased work of breathing. At first, her skin appeared to be slightly yellow. There were no dysmorphic features. At first it was difficult to pick up her saturations (pre- and post-ductal) due to her being so active. As she was not crying, the NIPE practitioner took the opportunity to auscultate her heart, finding her heart rate to be around 140 beats/min. There seemed to be a prominent impulse at the lower left sternal edge and, though it was difficult, the NIPE practitioner felt that there was a systolic murmur. Both the brachial and femoral pulses were felt equally. Her lung bases were clear and no liver could be felt.

Based on this, how concerned are you? How would you proceed? What would you say to Helen at this point?

The NIPE practitioner tried a different pulse oximetry machine and a Posi-Wrap, as well as asking Helen to hold Eve. The saturations read 75% in both the right hand and the foot, with a pulse corresponding to the auscultated apex rate. The paediatric registrar was fast bleeped to the examination room, who confirmed the findings. The doctor then trialled facial oxygen briefly, with no improvement in the saturations, and urgently admitted the baby to the neonatal unit. The baby was commenced on a prostaglandin infusion for a suspected duct-dependent cardiac defect. An echocardiogram was performed by a cardiologist who found severe stenosis of the pulmonary valve, with reduced blood flow across it, and a small duct, with blood flowing left to right. The baby improved with the prostaglandin, and went on to have cardiac surgery, making an excellent recovery.

What features were abnormal on the NIPE? How would you support, Helen, the mother, at the time of the urgent admission to the neonatal unit? What would you say to Helen, who is upset because she was told everything was normal on her antenatal scans?

analysis on the earlier UK PulseOx study (Ewer et al., 2011), involving six UK NHS trusts, screening 20,055 newborn infants, found that pulse oximetry as an adjunct to routine clinical examination was likely to be a cost-effective intervention (Roberts et al., 2012). Further cost-effectiveness data are currently being considered on the larger-scale UK study by Public Health England. Many NHS trusts are, however, currently undertaking newborn pulse oximetry before discharge. The timing of when the pulse oximetry is performed is variable because currently there is no national guidance.

As a NIPE practitioner, it is important to be aware of some of the caveats to performing pulse oximetry. It is important that any screening test does not lead to picking up a high number of falsely positive cases – in this case, not having congenital heart disease. However, a positive pulse oximetry screening test has been shown to pick up important non-cardiac conditions (e.g. pneumonia, early onset sepsis, pulmonary hypertension) in around 30–80% of cases that equally require urgent treatment (Ewer and Martin, 2016). It is also important to know that some cases of critical congenital heart disease are initially asymptomatic in the early stages (or may have mild cyanosis in an otherwise well infant [Plana et al., 2018]). Performing pulse oximetry early (i.e. before 24 hours of age) may pick up cases of critical congenital heart disease before an acute collapse, the latter having worse outcomes and greater risks of neurodevelopmental complications (Ewer, 2013).

It is also important to note that the post-ductal saturations should always be taken on the feet. Using the left hand may actually provide a false post-ductal reading because, in some infants, the duct inserts into the descending aorta at a similar place to the left subclavian artery, supplying blood to the left arm and hand.

CLINICAL TIP

The pre-ductal (right hand) should be the highest saturations. Avoid the left hand for post-ductal readings.

Ensure that a good tracing on both pre- and post-ductal saturations is obtained.

Referral for specialist opinion

As a NIPE practitioner, it is vital that, if you have any concerns about the cardio-vascular examination, the infant is reviewed in the early neonatal period by a senior paediatrician. If this is in the hospital setting, it is prudent that this review takes place before discharge. Below is a list of findings that would prompt such a review (Public Health England, 2018). The timing of such a review will depend on the underlying suspected condition, for example a murmur (with no other worrying features – see below) within the first 24 hours, with no other worrying features on examination or history, may need for be reviewed by a senior, once the infant has reached 24 hours of age. Any other clinical concerns would require a more urgent review (in the community, this would involve an urgent referral into the emergency department or your local paediatric service – it is important that community practitioners are aware of their referral pathways):

- Tachypnoea at rest
- Apnoea
- Respiratory distress (intercostal, subcostal, sternal, suprasternal recession, nasal flaring)
- Cyanosis, including failed pulse oximetry testing
- Visible pulsations over the praecordium – heaves, thrills
- Absent or weak femoral pulses
- Presence of a murmur or extra heart sounds
- Especially if loud, heard over a wide area, harsh quality.

Other features in the history that necessitate a review by a senior paediatrician, are:

- First-degree relative with critical congenital heart disease (especially coarc-tation of the aorta)

- Cardiac anomalies suspected on the antenatal scan
- Dysmorphic features on examination
- Concern about risk factors associated with congenital heart disease (see earlier in the chapter), especially if any clinical concerns.

It is important for all NIPE practitioners to remember that many infants will have a murmur in the first 24 hours of life without having a significant cardiac defect. However, the converse is also true: an infant with a significant cardiac defect requiring early intervention may not have an audible murmur. By following the above process, this is likely to be detected in the presence of other signs or a failed pulse oximetry screen. It is also important, after any NIPE examination, that parents are given clear advice on signs of illness or possible congenital heart disease to look out for (see above), the importance of having these reviewed as a matter of emergency and how to carry out such a medical review.

Resources on cardiovascular examination and congenital heart defects

There are several websites available for listening to heart sounds commonly found during the NIPE:

- https://med.stanford.edu/newborns/professional-education/photo-gallery/ heart.html

This is a very useful website to appreciate where to listen and the sounds for several different congenital heart defects, as well as normal heart sounds.

The internet is full of advice for parents on different aspects of congenital heart disease. As a NIPE practitioner it is imperative that you know where to direct parents to for reputable information. The British Heart Foundation is a useful source to direct parents to for an overview of congenital heart disease as well as information on specific defects: www.bhf.org.uk/heart-health/ conditions/congenital-heart-disease.

For all NIPE practitioners, it is important that we are aware of the national NIPE Programme standards and handbook. Signing up for the Public Health England blogs will provide you with all the relevant updated information on the NIPE Programme, as well as the other antenatal and newborn screening programmes that should be accessed as part of your continuing professional development: www.gov. uk/government/collections/newborn-and-infant-physical-examination-clinical-guidance

References

Askin, D. (2009). Fetal-to-neonatal transition: what is normal and what is not? Part 1. The physiology of transition. *Neonatal Network* **28**(3): 33–6.

Avery, G.B., MacDonald, M.G., Sesheia, M.K.M. and Mullett, M.D. (2005). *Avery's Neonatology. Pathology and Management of the Newborn*, 6th edn. London: LWW.

Bedford, C. and Lomax, A. (2015). *Examination of the Newborn: An Evidence-Based Guide*, 2nd edn. Chichester: Wiley Blackwell, pp. 32–61.

Blackburn, S.T. (2007). *Maternal, Fetal and Neonatal Physiology: A Clinical Perspective*, 3rd edn. St Louis, MO: Saunders.

Bohun, C.M., Potts, J.E., Casey, B.M. and Sandorm, G.G.S. (2007). A population-based study of cardiac malformations and outcomes associated with dextrocardia. *American Journal of Cardiology*, **100**: 305–9.

Ewer, A.K. (2013). Review of pulse oximetry screening for critical congenital heart defects in newborn infants. *Current Opinions in Cardiology*, **28**(2): 92–6.

Ewer, A.K., Martin, G.R. (2016). Newborn pulse oximetry screening: Which algorithm is best? *Pediatrics*, **138**(5): e20161206.

Ewer, A.K., Middleton, L.J., Furmston, A.T., Bhoyar, A., Daniels, J.P., Thangaratinam, S. et al. (2011). PulseOx Study Group Pulse oximetry screening for congenital heart defects in newborn infants (PulseOx): A test accuracy study. *The Lancet*, **378**(9793): 785–94.

Hoffmann, J.I. and Kaplan, S. (2002). The incidence of congenital heart disease. *Journal of the American College of Cardiology*, **39**: 1890–900.

Katzman, G.H. (1995). The newborn's SpO$_2$: a routine vital sign whose time has come? *Pediatrics*, **95**: 161–12.

Kenner, C. and Wright Lott, J. (2007). *Comprehensive Neonatal Care: An Interdisciplinary Approach*, 4th edn. London: Saunders.

Koppel, R.I., Druschel, C.M., Carter, T., Goldberg, B.E., Mehta, P.N., Talwar, R. and Bierman, F.Z. (2003). Effectiveness of pulse oximetry screening for congenital heart disease in asymptomatic newborns. *Pediatrics*, **111**: 451–5.

National Health Service Screening Programmes. (2015). Fetal Anomaly Screening Programme – Programme handbook, Available at: assets.publishing.service.gov.uk (accessed 11 May 2018).

Plana, M.N., Zamora, J., Suresh, G., Fernandez-Pineda, L., Thangaratinam, S. and Ewer, A.K. (2018). Pulse oximetry screening for critical congenital heart defects (Review). *Cochrane Database of Systematic Reviews*, 3: CD011912.

Public Health England (2018). Newborn and infant physical examination screening programme handbook. Section 5 – Examination of the heart. Available at: www.gov.uk/government/publications/newborn-and-infant-physical-examination-programme-handbook/newborn-and-infant-physical-examination-screening-programme-handbook#examination-of-the-heart.

Public Health England (2017). *PHE Screening* (online). Available at: https://phescreening.blog.gov.uk/2017/01/10/newborn-pulse-oximetry-pilot-update (accessed 28 May 2018).

Reich, J.D., Miller, S., Brogdon, B., Casatelli, J., Gompf, T.C., Huhta, J.C. and Sullivan, K. (2003). The use of pulse oximetry to detect congenital heart disease. *Journal of Pediatrics*, **142**: 268–72.

Rennie, J. (2012). *Rennie and Roberton's Textbook of Neonatology*, 5th edn. Edinburgh: Churchill Livingstone Elsevier, pp. 250–3.

Richmond, S., Reay, G. and Abu Harb, M. (2002). Routine pulse oximetry in the asymptomatic newborn. *Archives of Disease in Childhood: Fetal and Neonatal Edition*, **87**, F83–8.

Riede, F.T., Wörner, C., Dähnert, I., Möckel, A., Kostelka, M. and Schneider, P. (2010). Effectiveness of neonatal pulse oximetry screening for detection of critical congenital heart disease in daily clinical routine – results from a prospective multicenter study. *European Journal of Pediatrics*, **169**: 975–81.

Roberts, T.E., Barton, P.M., Auguste, P.E., Middleton, L.J., Furmston, A.T. and Ewer, AK. (2012). Pulse oximetry as a screening test for congenital heart defects in newborn infants: A cost-effectiveness analysis. *Archives of Disease in Childhood*, **97**: 221–6.

6C Examination of the respiratory system and the chest

Michelle Scott

The purpose of the examination of the chest and lungs is to identify any abnormalities. The role of the newborn infant physical examination (NIPE) practitioner is to differentiate normal variants from the abnormal and recognise when to refer for further review.

The respiratory examination starts with a thorough review of the maternal, antenatal and postnatal history (see Chapter 5), followed by careful physical examination. During the examination care must be taken to ensure that the baby is kept warm because cold stress will further exacerbate any respiratory symptoms (Polin and Spitzer, 2007). Physical examination of the respiratory system begins with careful visual and auditory observation, followed by auscultation and palpation. Clues to oxygen and respiratory status are most apparent at the observation stage of examination (Davies and McDonald, 2008). Cardinal signs of respiratory compromise, such as significant recession, tachypnoea and cyanosis, will require urgent senior colleague review and admission to the neonatal unit.

History taking before the examination

Table 6C.1 summarises important antenatal and postnatal considerations that could increase the risk of respiratory distress in the newborn (Tappero and Honeyfield, 2009).

There are often clues in the history that will aid decision-making if respiratory distress is present. For instance, transient tachypnoea of the newborn is more common in babies born by caesarean section (Al-Agha et al., 2010). Maternal risk factors for sepsis will increase the likelihood of congenital pneumonia or infection in the baby. Meconium-stained liquor increases the risk of meconium aspiration syndrome and, if the baby requires resuscitation at birth, use of positive pressure ventilation increases the risk of pneumothorax (Lissauer and Fanaroff, 2011).

Table 6C.1 History taking

Antenatal history	Postnatal history
• Maternal factors, i.e diabetes, sepsis, group B streptoccoci • Ultrasound findings ± neonatal alert form • Maternal medication/substance misuse • Prolonged rupture of the membranes and description, i.e. smell, clear • Meconium-stained Liquor • Gestational age • Delivery mode	• Apgar • Need for resuscitation • Age • Feeding • Signs of respiratory distress, i.e grunting • Apnoea

CLINICAL TIP

Assessment should include a history of the mother, infant and intrapartum issues.

Causes of respiratory distress in term infants

Table 6C.2 provides a summary of potential causes of respiratory distress in term infants.

Table 6.C2 Causes of respiratory distress in term infants

Common	Less common	Rare
• Transient tachypnoea of the newborn	• Pneumonia/sepsis • Meconium aspiration • Pneumothorax • Congenital heart disease/ heart failure • Persistent Pulmonary Hypertension of the Newborn • Hypoxic–ischaemic encephalopathy	• Surfactant deficiency • Diaphragmatic hernia • Tracheo-esophageal fistula • Pulmonary hypoplasia • Pleural effusion (chylothorax) • Milk aspiration • Airway obstruction, i.e choanal atresia • Lung abnormalities, i.e. cystic congenital adenomatoid malformation • Neuromuscular disorders • Severe anaemia • Metabolic acidosis (inborn error of metabolism)

Adapted from Lissauer and Fanaroff (2011).

Anatomy and physiology

The respiratory tract consists of the upper airway structures, including the nasal cavity, pharynx and larynx. The upper airways are heterogeneous and conduct a warm humidified airflow, but they do not participate in gaseous exchange. The lower airway consists of the intrathoracic trachea, bronchi, bronchioles and alveoli, and respiratory gas exchange occurs in portions of the respiratory bronchioles and alveolar ducts (Donn and Sinha, 2006).

The right lung consists of three lobes and the left two lobes. The pleural membrane encloses the lungs, and consists of an outer layer attached to the thoracic cavity (parietal pleura) and an inner layer that encapsulates the lung lobes (visceral pleura). Between the pleura and the lung is a fluid-filled cavity (Chamley et al., 2005).

The chest cavity is bounded by the sternum, 12 thoracic vertebrae and 12 pairs of ribs. The ribs in the neonate are more cartilaginous than in an adult, with incomplete ossification of the ribs. This accounts in part for the increased chest wall compliance in infants (Chamley et al., 2005). Below the ribs is the diaphragm, a thin flat layer of muscle that divides the thorax from the abdomen, and during quiet breathing is the primary muscle for ventilation (Donn and Sinha, 2006).

Other palpable thoracic landmarks include the suprasternal notch and the xiphoid process, which are found on the upper and lower aspects of the sternum. The clavicles and scapulae complete the bony structure of the chest (Figure 6C.1).

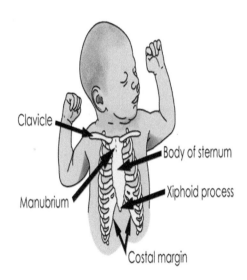

Figure 6C.1
Neonatal bony structures

Before birth, the lungs are fluid filled and gas exchange occurs via the placenta. As the fetus is squeezed through the birth canal, the fetal thoracic cavity is compressed, expelling much of this fluid. Some fluid remains, however, but is rapidly absorbed by the body shortly after birth. The first inhalation occurs within 10 seconds after birth and not only serves as the first inspiration, but also acts to inflate the lungs (Resuscitation Council UK, 2016).

Pulmonary surfactant is a naturally occurring substance critical for inflation to occur, because it reduces the surface tension of the alveoli. It is produced late in the second trimester and early third trimester, and deficiency causes respiratory distress syndrome. Antenatal corticosteroids promote surfactant synthesis and lung maturation. Although the predominant risk factor for respiratory distress syndrome is preterm delivery, other risk factors are maternal diabetes, infection, hypoxaemia, acidaemia and hypothermia (Donn and Sinha, 2006; Lissauer and Fanaroff, 2011).

Reference lines

It is useful to be able to identify the location of any examination findings to provide an accurate description for the medical notes or to a senior colleague when requesting a review (Figure 6C.2 and Table 6C.3).

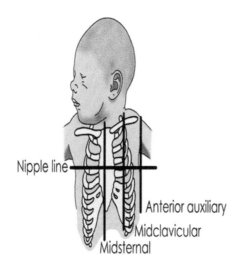

Figure 6C.2
Reference lines

Table 6C.3 Reference lines

1 Nipple line	Refers to a horizontal line through the nipples
2 Anterior axillary line	Extends vertically from the anterior axillary fold
3 Midclavicular line	Vertical line from the middle of the clavicle
4 Midsternal line	A vertical line through the body of the sternum

Visual inspection

Before physical examination, the practitioner should take a few moments to observe the baby for signs of respiratory distress. This should ideally be while the baby is quiet and relaxed. Does the baby look ill or well? Consideration of colour, respiratory rate, work of breathing, tone and activity can all provide clues to the oxygen and respiratory status of the baby.

Colour

Observe the colour of the infant's skin. Lips and mucous membranes should be pink and well perfused. If cyanosis is present, it is important to differentiate peripheral cyanosis, which is relatively common, from central cyanosis, which is potentially serious.

Peripheral cyanosis

Peripheral cyanosis or acrocyanosis describes a blue or purple colour of the hands and/or feet. It is common immediately after birth or when the baby is cold. It is usually seen in the first 24 hours of life and is not a reflection of hypoxaemia (Baston and Durward, 2017). When peripheral cyanosis occurs with normal oxygen saturations and good central perfusion (capillary refill time <2 seconds), offer an explanation to the parents and advise them to keep the baby warm. If the infant is poorly perfused centrally, ask for a further review because the infant may require management of suspected sepsis (Polin and Spitzer, 2007).

Central cyanosis

When a baby is centrally cyanosed, the remainder of the body will have a blue discoloration including the lips, the mucous membrane of the mouth and the tongue. Cyanosis is a relatively late sign of respiratory distress and does not develop until the oxygen saturation drops to 75% or less (Polin and Spitzer, 2007). Causes of central cyanosis include congenital heart disease, infection, neuromuscular disorders or underlying respiratory disease. The infant will have low oxygen saturations, and will need supplemental oxygen administration and urgent neonatal review because admission to the neonatal unit will be required.

Tone

Observe the baby's muscle tone and levels of activity. Tone after birth is usually a flexed curled position. Movement should be symmetrical, with both arms and legs moving equally when awake. Hypotonia or inactivity is concerning and may indicate an underlying pathology. In the absence of good muscle tone, the tongue can fall back against the soft palate and obstruct the airway (Tappero and Honeyfield, 2009).

Rate and pattern

The normal respiratory rate for a newborn infant is around 30–60 breaths/min with wide variations. Respirations are usually quiet, and chest movement symmetrical and without recession. Abdominal breathing is normal due to the diaphragm being the primary muscle of respiration. The normal breathing pattern is irregular and will vary according to temperature, sleep and after feeding (Baston and Durward, 2017).

Babies delivered by caesarean section may have an increased respiratory rate in the first 24 hours due to the increased likelihood of retaining fetal lung fluid, when compared with those born vaginally. This should settle within the first 2 hours of life.

Recession

The chest wall of the newborn is very compliant. Recession is the term used to describe indrawing of the chest wall on inspiration, in an attempt to generate high intrathoracic pressures to ventilate poorly compliant lungs (Donn and Sinha, 2006). Recession is described according to the location and may be intercostal (in between the ribs), subcostal (below the chest wall) or sternal recession (Figure 6C.3).

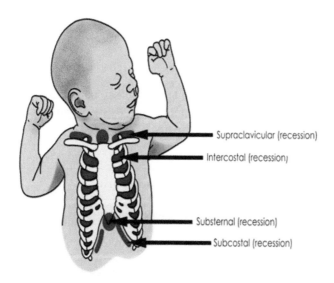

Figure 6C.3
Neonatal chest and recession

Respiratory muscles fatigue when the work of breathing is increased, strength is reduced or inefficiency results. Clinical manifestations of respiratory muscle fatigue include progressive hypercapnia and apnoea (Donn and Sinha, 2006).

Apnoea

Apnoea is defined as a pause in breathing in excess of 20 seconds and is often accompanied by slowing of the heart rate (bradycardia). In the preterm population, self-correcting bradycardias and transient apnoeas are not uncommon due to immaturity of respiratory control mechanisms. In the term or near-term infant, apnoea is abnormal and may be a result of underlying pathology (Lissauer and Fanaroff, 2011) (Table 6C.4). Apnoeic infants require immediate medical attention.

> **THINK POINT**
>
> Consider the signs of respiratory compromise that you have witnessed in clinical practice were they obvious?

Grunting

Grunting is the sound made as the infant breathes out against a partially closed glottis to prevent airway collapse during expiration. It typically occurs in transient tachypnoea of the newborn, pneumonia and respiratory distress syndrome (Donn and Sinha 2006).

Nasal flaring

Babies are mainly nose breathers. During nasal flaring, the nostrils widen during inspiration. Immediately following delivery mild nasal flaring is common but should settle within the first 1–2 hours.

Table 6C.4 Causes of apnoea in the newborn

- Exhaustion after a period of recession and tachypnoea
- Sepsis
- Hypoglycaemia
- Seizure
- Central nervous system abnormality, i.e intracranial haemorrhage, neuromuscular disorders, drug withdrawal

Polin and Spitzer (2007).

THINK POINT

The differential diagnosis for neonatal respiratory distress is very broad.

Chest shape

A newborn infant's chest is rounded rather than flattened, as seen in older children (Chamley et al., 2005).

Asymmetry: chest movement is usually symmetrical. Asymmetrical chest movement may be a result of a pneumothorax, diaphragmatic hernia or congenital heart disease.

Hyperinflation: the chest appears barrel shaped and may be associated with diaphragmatic hernia, or air trapping due to meconium aspiration syndrome or transient tachypnoea of the newborn.

Pectus excavatum: this is the term used to describe a chest where the sternum appears indented or funnel shaped. Usually, there is no clinical concern but it can be associated with Marfan's and Noonan's syndromes.

Pectus carinatum: the sternum protrudes outwards and is rarely clinically significant but it may be associated with Marfan's and Noonan's syndromes (Tappero and Honeyfield, 2009).

Breast engorgement: due to the effects of maternal oestrogen some babies may have breasts that are engorged or enlarged. This usually lasts no more than a week and is of no clinical significance.

Nipples: look for number, placement and spacing. Widely spaced nipples may be indicative of Turner's syndrome and the baby may require bloods taken for chromosomal analysis. Accessory nipples may be located anywhere on the vertical nipple line and an outpatient department referral may be made to discuss management options.

CLINICAL TIP

An indrawn or sunken abdomen is referred to as a scaphoid abdomen and can be a symptom of a diaphragmatic hernia (where the abdominal contents have herniated into the chest cavity).

Secretions: secretions are often evident during transition; sometimes the appearance of oral and nasal secretions is in an attempt to clear fetal lung fluid. Normal secretions are clear. Oral secretions may also evidence contents swallowed during the birth. Excessive oral secretions may be indicative of oesophageal atresia and nasal stuffiness may be associated with maternal drug use or congenital syphilis (Polin and Spitzer, 2007).

Physical examination

Auscultation

Breath sounds are louder and coarser in the newborn when compared with an adult due to infants having less subcutaneous tissue.

Using a warmed paediatric stethoscope, listen for the presence and equality of breath sounds on both sides during inspiration and expiration. Start at the top and move systematically from side to side listening to six areas, including the upper, middle and lower part of the chest in a '2' shape (Davies and McDonald, 2008) (Figure 6C.4). Auscultation of breaths sounds via the midaxilla, around the sixth intercostal space and on the back, will most adequately assess the lower lobes. Practitioners should be able to hear the respiratory rate clearly as a soft of muffled sound and there should be no extra sounds.

A reduction in air entry is usually heard with severe lung disease (i.e. respiratory distress syndrome) and a unilateral decrease in air entry may be heard in any unilateral lung disease (i.e. pneumonia, pneumothorax) (Donn and Sinha, 2006).

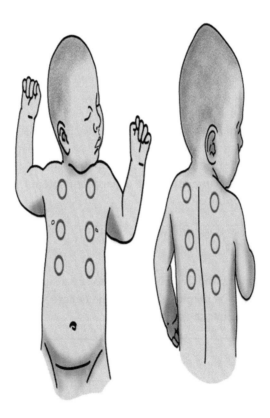

Figure 6C.4
Drawing of the sequential placement of stethoscope for chest auscultation

Adventitious sounds

Localisation of adventitious breath sounds may be difficult due to the small size of the chest.

Bowel sounds: these can occasionally be heard over the lung fields. They may be referred sounds transmitted from the abdomen or due to a diaphragmatic hernia. If bowel sounds are heard during lung auscultation, a member of the neonatal team should be asked to review the baby.

Crackles, râles or crepitations: these are discrete, discontinuous, brief cracking or bubbling sounds.

Fine crackles can be simulated by rubbing together a lock of hair. They are most often heard in the first few hours of life and are also associated with respiratory distress syndrome.

Medium crackles are similar to the sound of a fizzy drink. And are associated with pneumonia or transient tachypnoea of the newborn.

Coarse crackles are loud and bubbly and are associated with significant mucus or fluid in the large airways (Donn and Sinha, 2006; Tappero and Honeyfield, 2009).

Rhonchus: this is best described as a loud, low coarse sound resembling a snore and may be heard at any point during inspiration or expiration. It is associated with secretions and often heard after a caesarean section or when there is meconium aspiration (Donn and Sinha, 2006; Tappero and Honeyfield, 2009).

Stridor: this is a high-pitched, hoarse sound usually during inspiration at the larynx or upper airways. The presence of a stridor may indicate partial obstruction of the airways and should be referred to the neonatal team for prompt further investigation (Polin and Spitzer, 2007).

Wheezes: these are due to air moving through a narrowed airway. It is a high-pitched, squeaking, continuous sound that may be louder during expiration. Wheezing is rarely heard in the newborn (Tappero and Honeyfield, 2009).

Palpation

After inspection and auscultation of breath sounds, areas of the chest should be palpated by the examiner during the routine newborn examination.

Clavicle

The clavicle is the bone most commonly fractured during delivery and should be checked as part of the postnatal examination. A fractured clavicle is most likely to occur in large babies who have had a difficult delivery (Laroia, 2008). Signs that the clavicle may be fractured include asymmetrical movement of the arms and an incomplete Moro's reflex may also be present on the affected side (Baston and Durward, 2017). On examination, it is important to palpate the entire length of both clavicles to the shoulder joint for any irregularity. If crepitus, swelling or tenderness is present, suspect a fracture (Flannigan, 2011). If there are concerns that the clavicle may be fractured, a chest radiograph should be ordered to confirm the diagnosis. Fractures will generally heal quickly in around 7–10 days without any intervention. Paracetamol may be prescribed on an as-required basis for pain. Outpatient department follow-up should be arranged (Flannigan, 2011).

THINK POINT

If you suspect a fractured clavicle during a NIPE, how would you explain this to a parent?

Breast tissue

Breast tissue should be palpated to determine masses, secretions, fissures or hypertrophy. Breast swelling can occur in both male and female babies. Breast engorgement may be due to the effects of maternal oestrogen; some babies may have breasts that are engorged or enlarged. This usually lasts no more than a week and is of no clinical significance. Occasionally, there may be a white discharge from the nipple and this is usually self-resolving (Flannigan, 2011).

Erythema, tenderness and increased temperature over a swelling may indicate an abscess, and the baby will need to be referred to the neonatal team for investigations, antibiotics and possible surgical opinion (Flannigan, 2011; Baston and Durward, 2017).

Sternum and ribs: palpate for crepitus or masses. The tip of the xiphoid process often protrudes anteriorly and may move with pressure.

Pulse oximetry

Pulse oximetry is a simple non-invasive test that can measure, the amount of oxygen carried around the body by red blood cells using a sensor placed on the newborn infant's hand or foot. Pulse oximetry measures the relative absorption of light by saturated and unsaturated haemoglobin, which absorbs light at different frequencies (Donn and Sinha, 2006). Normal oxygen saturations should be between 95% and 100%. Cyanosis often does not develop until the oxygen saturation drops to 75% or less in a full-term infant, so hypoxaemia may be unrecognised in the absence of other clinical signs (Polin and Spitzer, 2007).

CLINICAL TIP

Respiratory symptoms may be a symptom of an underlying cardiac abnormality.

Transillumination

A bright light source is applied to the chest wall and can be a useful adjunct to the physical examination when a pneumothorax is suspected. To be effective, the light source has to be extremely bright and the area around the baby dark. The procedure should be performed only by a senior member of the neonatal team.

Upper airway disorders

Choanal atresia: this is a rare bony obstruction between the nasal cavity and the nasopharynx. If bilateral, there will be respiratory distress and cyanosis due to airway obstruction because newborn infants are obligatory nose breathers. Colour will improve when crying or when the mouth is opened. Choanal atresia will require surgical correction (Lissauer and Fanaroff, 2011).

Pierre Robin sequence: this describes a sequence of abnormalities including:

- Micrognathia (small jaw)
- Posteriorly displaced tongue
- Cleft palate.

There may be other anomalies, particularly congenital heart disease. The most serious complication is respiratory obstruction.

End of chapter quiz

1 At what level of desaturation is cyanosis detectable at physical examination in most infants?
2 Are infants of mothers with diabetes at more or less risk of developing signs of respiratory distress?
3 What are significant signs of respiratory distress in the newborn?
4 Explain the difference between pectus carinatum and pectus excavatum and what conditions they may be associated with.
5 Why is it important to keep the baby warm during the NIPE examination?

References

Al-Aghaa, A., Kinsley, B.T., Finucanea, F.M., Murray, S., Daly, S., Foley, M. et al. (2010). Caesarean section and macrosomia increase transient tachypnoea of the newborn in type 1 diabetes pregnancies. *Diabetes Research and Clinical Practice*, **89**(3): 46–8.

Baston, H. and Durward, H. (2017). *Examination of the Newborn. A Practical Guide*, 3rd edn. London: Routledge.

Chamley, C.A., Carson, P., Randall, D. and Sandwell, M. (2005). *Developmental Anatomy and Physiology of Children. A Practical Approach*. Edinburgh: Elsevier Churchill Livingstone.

Davies, L. and McDonald, S. (2008). *Examination of the Newborn and Neonatal Health: A Multidimensional Approach*. Edinburgh: Churchill Livingstone.

Donn, S.M. and Sinha, S.K. (2006). *Manual of Neonatal Respiratory Care*, 2nd edn. Philadelphia, PA: Elsevier.

Flannigan, C. (2011). *A Practical Guide to Managing Paediatric Problems on the Postnatal Wards*. Oxford: Radcliffe Publishing.

Laroia, N. (2008). Birth trauma. *Emedicine*. Available at: http://emedicine.medscape.com/article/980112-overview.

Lissauer, T. and Fanaroff, A.A. (2011). *Neonatology at a Glance*, 2nd edn. Chichester: Wiley-Blackwell.

Polin, R.A. and Spitzer, A.R. (2007). *Fetal and Neonatal Secrets*, 2nd edn. Philadelphia, PA: Elsevier.

Resuscitation Council UK (2016). *Newborn Life Support*, 4th edn. London: Resuscitation Council UK.

Tappero, E.P. and Honeyfield, M.E. (2009). *Physical Assessment of the Newborn. A Comprehensive Approach to the Art of Physical Examination*, 4th edn. Petaluma, PA: NICU Ink Book Publishers.

D Examination of the newborn abdomen and genitalia

Natalie Fairhurst

Introduction

The aim of this chapter is not to create an expert on every finding in relation to the newborn abdomen and genitalia, but rather to educate on different variations of normal, congenital anomalies that may be identified antenatally or postnatally on examination, and when to refer to a senior colleague for review. Alongside this, a practical guide is available on the technique of abdominal examination.

There are several purposes that highlight the importance of the abdominal and genitalia examination. For most, it will simply be clarification of normality for both the examiner and the parents, providing reassurance for medically insignificant findings that may worry the parents. If an abnormality were to be found, it should lead to prompt referral to the appropriate professional or team, resulting in timely management and improved outcome. Finally, one of the four key components of the newborn infant physical examination (NIPE) examination, inspection of the testes, is included in this part of the examination.

History taking before the examination

Communication with the family is vital and there are several pertinent questions that the parents should be asked, in addition to reviewing the antenatal history from the maternal notes, to allow a holistic assessment of the abdomen. The information collected should be used as a guide while undertaking the examination.

Antenatal history

- Check antenatal scan reports and communicate with the parents about any findings such as cysts, abdominal masses, renal abnormalities or echogenicity within the bowel or liver.

- Review the maternal notes and discuss with the midwife caring for the mother and infant with regard to any antenatal plan that may have been made.
- Ask the parents if there is any family history of abdominal, genitalia or renal problems from birth, in the immediate family, because there is a strong connection between previous family history and congenital anomalies.

Discussion of the antenatal history will heighten your awareness of any abnormalities that might be found during the examination. This will allow a prompt senior referral, a treatment plan and any required further investigations. Be aware of whether the family have been seen antenatally and that there was a confirmed risk, because then a clear plan should be available and your only action may be to refer for senior review. Remember, even if this is the case, you will need to offer appropriate support, and communication to the family.

Feeding history

A detailed feeding history includes:

- How is the infant feeding? By bottle, breast, syringe or cup?
- What type of milk is the infant being fed? Breast milk or formula?
- How often is the infant feeding and what volumes are they taking?
- Is the infant vomiting? If so, is it milky, contains blood (fresh or old) or bilious (yellow or green)?
- Has the infant passed urine in the first 24 hours of life?
- If a male infant, did he have a normal urine stream?
- Has the infant had their bowels opened in the first 48 hours of life?

A detailed history in combination with a thorough examination will allow a holistic assessment of the current state of the infant. Once a history has been established it should be mentally referred too throughout the examination.

Bilious vomiting in the newborn requires an immediate senior referral and continued assessment. It should be considered as a possible bowel obstruction, such as a malrotation with volvulus, until proven otherwise (Blackburn, 2015). Significant abdominal distension and failure to pass meconium within the first 48 hours both warrant a senior review and compliance with local guidelines initiated in a timely manner.

Visual inspection of the newborn abdomen

Before commencement of palpation of the abdomen or a physical examination of any other part of the infant, a visual inspection should be conducted. This will allow assessment of many aspects such as colour, shape and any immediately noted abnormality while the infant is in a restful state.

The abdominal colour should be in keeping with the rest of the infant's natural skin tone. It should not be dusky or discoloured. The abdomen may look slightly full, particularly after a feed, but should not be distended. A normal finding that may be observed is diastasis recti. This presents as a linear bulge down the centre of the abdomen due to weakness in the abdominal muscle. It requires no intervention and will resolve spontaneously over time (Stanford Children's Health, 2017).

CLINICAL TIP

Bilious vomiting, abdominal distension and/or non-passage of meconium within 48 hours requires urgent senior review.

Umbilicus

The umbilical cord will have been cut and clamped at delivery. It may vary in thickness and length between babies.

Vessels

The umbilical cord should contain two arteries and one vein, which will be encased in Wharton's jelly. It is the role of the midwife to examine the cord and placenta after birth, including counting of the vessels (Harris, 2011) because the presence of only one artery can be associated with other congenital anomalies (Gimovsky et al., 2018). Once the cord has been clamped this inspection can become difficult.

Hernia

Umbilical hernias are very common in newborn babies (Cincinatti Children's, 2016). A hernia will appear when some fatty tissue or bowel protrudes through a weakening in the muscle wall. Of umbilical hernias 80–90% will close spontaneously and do not require an immediate referral; however, parents should be advised to seek immediate help if the hernia changes in appearance or their infant is in pain or distress, begins vomiting or becomes constipated.

An infant may also present with a hernia in the groin called an inguinal hernia. These can present in both males and females. There is a risk of the bowel becoming stuck in the inguinal canal, resulting in damage due a decreased blood supply, so these hernias do require a senior referral.

Omphalitis

Omphalitis is an infection of the umbilical stump (Gallagher et al., 2017). Risk factors include an unplanned homebirth, maternal sepsis, low birth weight, prolonged rupture of the membranes and chorioamnionitis (Stewart and Benitz,

2016). Although these risk factors are commonly seen in practice, omphalitis is rare, affecting around 1 in 1000 babies (Stewart and Benitz, 2016). It presents as a superficial cellulitis on the abdominal wall surrounding the umbilical stump, which may quickly spread and worsen (Gallagher et al., 2017). Identification should prompt referral to local guidelines for treatment.

Physical examination of the newborn abdomen

Technique for palpation

On palpation the infant needs to be relaxed with the abdomen fully exposed, but also kept as warm as possible. Ensure that your hands are warm. The abdomen should be soft and easy to palpate. A firm or tender abdomen is a cause for concern because it could be an indication of several bowel problems such as a perforation or an obstruction.

1   Using the flats of your index, middle and third finger, commence the examination in the lower part of the groin. It could be possible that the infant has significant organ enlargement so, if you palpate above the groin, you may miss this.
2   Using a sweeping motion, keeping your fingers in contact with the abdomen at all times, gradually work your way up until you reach the subcostal region.
3   Perform this on both the left and the right sides of the abdomen in turn.

Palpation should be easy if the abdomen is soft. The infant is likely to react to this part of the examination, usually through being active and tensing the abdomen, so it may be useful to have a parent or colleague assist by allowing the infant to suck on a dummy, if supplied by parents, or a gloved finger. Focused attention should apply when palpating both sides of the abdomen. Although rare, an infant may be born with situs inversus – a condition in which the internal organs are reversed and therefore may be palpated on the opposite sides.

> ## CLINICAL TIP
>
> A parent is likely to be more than willing to talk to their infant while letting them suck on their finger to keep them calm, so do not be afraid to ask the parent to help!

Liver

The identification of a liver edge does not always indicate a problem. Hepatomegaly in newborns is defined as a liver edge more than 3.5 cm below the right subcostal margin (University of Chicago, 2013). However, it is important to remember that the liver can also be displaced, for example if the infant has a pneumothorax, a mass, cyst or abscess may also present as hepatomegaly (Wolf and Lavine, 2000). Despite this, all of these cases would require referral to a senior member of staff.

Spleen

One-third of newborns may have a palpable spleen tip that may be felt less than 1–2 cm below the left costal margin (Gozman, 2017). Enlargement of the spleen is usually found together with liver enlargement known as hepatosplenomegaly. One of the most common causes to be considered is TORCH infections, whether TORCH stands for **to**xoplasmosis, **r**ubella, **c**ytomegalovirus (CMV) and **h**erpes simplex virus (HSV). A thorough maternal history and referral to a senior colleague are vital for diagnosis.

Kidneys

Kidneys can be balloted to determine their presence and size by placing one hand on the infant's back, the other on the abdomen and gently palpating downwards. If you are concerned about your findings then always request a senior review.

Examination of the newborn genitalia

Again, as with the abdomen, a visual inspection of the genitalia should be performed before the physical examination (Table 6D.1). Many abnormalities can

Table 6D.1 Genitalia findings	
Male	Female
Cryptorchidism (undescended testes)	White/blood-tinged discharge
Retractile testes	Labial fusion/adhesion
Hypospadias	Hymenal skin tags
Chordee	Ambiguous genitalia
Hydrocele	
Micropenis	
Inguinal hernia	
Partial foreskin development	
Testicular torsion	
Ambiguous genitalia	

be noted simply from a visual inspection; however, some may be found only during a physical examination.

Physical examination of the testes

Technique for palpation

As with the abdominal examination, clean warm hands are a necessity. If not already undressed, the infant will need to be exposed from the waist down, including full removal of the nappy. A visual inspection will have already been done, thereby alerting the examiner to any immediate abnormality.

1   Each testicle needs individual palpation. Using the thumb and index finger, gently palpate the scrotum to feel the whole testicle.
2   If the testicle cannot be felt then the examiner must attempt to milk the testicle down from the inguinal canal. This can be done by gently pressing the thumb from the top of the groin and slowly sliding downwards, feeling for the testicle as the scrotum is reached.
3   Upon completion of the examination, the hands must be washed and dried before continuing.

The four outcomes of the examination of the testes are discussed below.

Male

Testes

There are four findings that are possible after examination of the testes. These are:

1   Normal, both testes are descended into the scrotum
2   Two testes are palpable but either one or both are retractile or in the inguinal canal
3   Unilateral undescended testis
4   Bilateral undescended testes.

Public Health England (2016) provides clear guidance as to the management for each finding.

> ## THINK POINT
>
> Testes are one of the four key components of the NIPE. What are the other three?

Screen negative

If no abnormality is detected during the examination, then no further follow-up is required. Parents should simply advised be to seek help if they have any concerns about their infant's testes.

Screen positive

If either one or both testes are found to be impalpable, or are not in the correct position, the actions required are:

1 Unilateral undescended testis: to be reviewed at the second examination at 6–8 weeks (see Chapter 9).
2 Bilateral undescended testes: to be reviewed by a senior paediatrician or neonatologist within 24 hours to rule out any metabolic or intersex conditions.

Scrotum

The size of the scrotum can be an immediate visual indicator as to whether the testes have descended. In undescended testes the scrotum will appear small. Rugosities (wrinkles) should be visualised on the scrotum. A large smooth scrotum can be an indicator of a hydrocele, which is an accumulation of fluid around one or both testes.

Transillumination technique

A hydrocele can be confirmed by transillumination. By holding a light at the base of the scrotum, shining upwards, it can be confirmed whether the area is fluid filled (by the light shining through) or if there is a mass, such as an incarcerated testicle (light will be blocked and show a darkened area).

There is the external skin of the scrotum has an area of discoloration such as erythema or darkening, a testicular torsion should be considered. Other signs may present such as tenderness and a firm testicle. This is a time-sensitive surgical emergency and requires an immediate senior review and surgical referral.

Position of urinary meatus

The urinary meatus should be positioned at the tip of the head of the penis. In some boys, the meatus may be positioned in one of several places on the genitalia known as hypospadias. There are four classifications of the position of the meatus (Figure 6D.1).

There are other problems that are associated with hypospadias such as chordee, a downward curvature of the penis, and the abnormal development of the foreskin resulting in a hood-like structure. A senior review will be

Glanular   Midshaft   Penoscrotal   Perineal

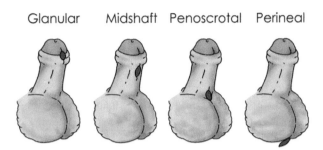

Figure 6D.1
Four classifications of hypospadias

required facilitating a urology referral. The urine stream should be observed and reported to urology during the referral process. Parents should be advised to withhold from circumcising their infant until he has been seen by the urologist.

Shape and size of penis

The normal length of a newborn penis is between 2.8 and 4.2 cm (1.1–1.6 inches) (Stanford Children's Health, 2017). Although not done routinely, when measuring the size of the penis, the base should be identified and measured up to the tip. Micropenis would be defined as a penis length less than 1.9 cm (Stanford Children's Health, 2017). This can be an isolated finding but is also associated with various hormonal disorders. The penis should be straight, but, as mentioned above, an infant may be noted to have chordee. Although chordee is associated with hypospadias, it can also be an isolated finding.

Female

Appearance

Whether the infant is examined soon after birth or several days later may have an impact on the immediate appearance of the vagina. Soon after birth it may still appear red and swollen. A reduced gestational age can also result in more prominent looking labia minora and clitoris.

Labia

The labia majora and minora should both be parted to ensure that there is no labial fusion/adhesion and that the vaginal opening is patent. If the labia cannot be parted, either fully or partially, or a vaginal opening is not visualised, then a senior review is required.

A hymenal skin tag may be observed to be slightly protruding from the vaginal opening. This is a normal finding and should reduce within 4–6 weeks' time. No referral is required.

Discharge

Newborn girls may have a thick mucous discharge, sometimes blood stained, due to maternal oestrogen stimulation of the vaginal mucosa, cervical epithelium and endometrium (Hann and Fertleman, 2016). This may last around 7–10 days. Parents should be reassured that this is normal.

Disorders of sexual development

Disorders of sexual development (DSDs) are when the reproductive organs and genitalia do not develop in the expected way (Houk et al., 2018). There are many variations of DSDs and this is too broad of a topic to be covered in great detail here. Below are some examples of the more common disorders that you may come across when undertaking a newborn examination.

Ambiguous genitalia

The presence of ambiguous genitalia can signal a potentially life-threatening disorder (Krishnan and Wisniewski, 2015), and therefore requires prompt identification, review and management. Attentiveness to normal male and female genitalia is consequently required.

There are several characteristics that may be observed when identifying whether genitalia may be ambiguous (Table 6D.2).

Table 6D.2 Characteristics of ambiguous genitalia

Male	Female
Hypospadias	Enlarged clitoris (or what may be a small penis)
An unusually small penis	Absence of vaginal opening
Absence of both testes	Palpable testes in what appears to be the labia majora
Smooth scrotum with no rugae	
Indentation/opening down centre of what appears to be the scrotum	

Congenital adrenal hyperplasia

Congenital adrenal hyperplasia (CAH) can be present at birth (congenital) with larger than usual adrenal glands (adrenal hyperplasia). In CAH, an enzyme is missing from the body, resulting in an impaired ability to release the hormone *cortisol* (Great Ormond Street Hospital, 2015). This, in turn, increases the amount of *androgens* produced, causing early symptoms for boys and ambiguous genitalia for girls. Table 6D.3 shows some of the early symptoms of CAH.

Due to the potential 'salt-losing crisis' that can occur with CAH, an urgent senior review is required to allow initiation of appropriate investigations and possible referral to the local endocrinology team.

Alongside CAH there are many other reasons for ambiguous genitalia in both boys and girls that may need referral to endocrinology, so all cases will need urgent senior review.

Anus

The anus should be carefully inspected for both presence and tone. The exact cause of anorectal malformations (ARMs) is not known and they are more commonly associated with chromosomal abnormalities. The incidence is between 1 in 2000 and 1 in 5000 live births (Gangopadhyay et al., 2015). They can easily be missed without thorough inspection and with early identification long-term outcomes can be improved (Weledji et al., 2016). There are several types of anorectal anomalies that can involve the anus, rectum or both. Any abnormal anal findings should be referred to a senior colleague for review and referral.

CLINICAL TIP

The presence of meconium in the nappy does not rule out an anorectal malformation.

Table 6D.3 Early symptoms of congenital adrenal hyperplasia

Male	Female
Vomiting	Virilised (male-appearing) genitalia
Dehydration	Hyponatraemia
Hyponatraemia	
Abnormal heart rhythms	
Hypoglycaemia	

Anal stenosis

Anal stenosis is when the anal opening is present and in the correct place, but is noted to be smaller than normal. Although a relatively common finding in neonates, if missed this can result in rectal perforation (Khan et al., 2015).

Anterior ectopic anus

An ectopic anus is when there is a small opening but in the wrong place. The opening is usually anteriorly placed on the perineum. The passing of meconium can be falsely reassuring of a normal anus. Newborn meconium is soft and can pass easily through even a small opening.

Imperforate anus

An imperforate anus is where there is no anal opening at all. In some cases, although the anal opening is absent, a girl may have a rectovestibular or rectovaginal fistula, resulting in passage of meconium, parallel to or through the vagina, and a boy may have a rectourethral fistula, thereby passing meconium through the urethral meatus.

There are other serious and potentially life-threatening clinical conditions that can present at the newborn examination. Gastrointestinal pathology, including a trachea-oesophageal fistula, distended abdomen with bile-stained vomiting, an imperforate anus, or a suspected one, all require an urgent senior paediatrician review and transfer to the neonatal unit. After stabilisation and diagnostic investigation, these conditions require onward transfer to a tertiary neonatal surgical unit.

End of chapter quiz

1   Why is it important to have a thorough history alongside a comprehensive examination?
2   How can a hydrocele be differentiated from, for example, a testicular torsion?
3   Why may a newborn girl have blood-tinged discharge?
4   What condition can result in a 'salt-losing crisis' in both boys and girls?
5   Does the passing of meconium confirm a normal anus?

References

Blackburn, S. (2015). Term newborns with bilious vomiting: When should they see a surgeon and how soon? *Archives of Diseases in Childhood*, **100**(1): 1–2.
Cincinatti Children's (2016). Umbilical hernia (online) Available at: www.cincinnatichildrens.org/health/u/umbilical-hernia (accessed 5 September 2018).

Gallagher, P.G., Zanelli, S.A. and Shah, S (2017). Omphalitis (online) Available at: https://emedicine.medscape.com/article/975422-overview?pa=yLU%2BwJj0XOa iDQGqmEZWL2%2BXrC9WMIq2wZmTb2aIQGHEKf5E7mK7npbXxvpHZAfEwy p7aOVXd4gIncY%2B24N3OichrzF%2F7vlnSF6AEX%2F09M8%3D (accessed 18 February 2018).

Gangopadhyay, A. and Panday, V. (2015). Anorectal malformations. *Journal of Indian Association of Paediatric Surgeons*, **20**(1): 10–15.

Gimovsky, M., Tejero Rosa, E. and Sepulvelda, W (2018). Single umbilical artery. *Up To Date* (online). Available at: www.uptodate.com/contents/single-umbilical-artery (accessed 27 March 2018).

Gozman, A. (2017). Pediatric splenomegaly (online). Available at: https://emedicine. medscape.com/article/958739-overview (accessed 11 February 2018).

Great Ormond Street Hospital (2015). Congenital adrenal hyperplasia (online). Available at: www.gosh.nhs.uk/conditions-and-treatments/conditions-we-treat/ congenital-adrenal-hyperplasia (accessed 31 March 2018).

Hann, G. and Fertleman, C. (2016). *The Child Protection Practice Manual*. Oxford: Oxford University Press.

Harris, J. (2011). How to perform an examination of the placenta. *Midwives Magazine* (online). Available at: www.rcm.org.uk/news-views-and-analysis/analysis/ how-to%E2%80%A6-perform-an-examination-of-the-placenta (accessed 27 February 2018).

Houk, C., Baskin, L. and Levitsky, L. (2018). Management of the infant with atypical genitalia (disorder of sex development) (online). Available at: www.uptodate. com/contents/management-of-the-infant-with-atypical-genitalia-disorder-of-sex-development (accessed 5 September 2018).

Khan, A.R., Malik, A. and Aslam, A. (2015). Neonatal rectal perforation: rare complication of congenital anal stenosis. *Journal of Paediatric Surgical Specialities*, **9**(2): 1–52.

Krishnan, S. and Wisniewski, A. (2015). Ambiguous genitalia in the newborn. *Endotext* (online). Available at: www.ncbi.nlm.nih.gov/books/NBK279168 (accessed 31 March 2018).

Public Health England (2016). Newborn and infant physical examination screening programme handbook (online). Available at: www.gov.uk/government/uploads/ system/uploads/attachment_data/file/572685/NIPE_programme_handbook_ 2016_to_2017_November_2016.pdf (accessed 27 March 2018).

Stanford Children's Health (2017). Abdomen (online). Available at: https://med. stanford.edu/newborns/professional-education/photo-gallery/abdomen.html (accessed 11 February 2018).

Stewart, D. and Benitz, W. (2016). Umbilical cord care in the newborn infant. *Pediatrics*, **138**(3): e1–5.

University of Chicago (2013). Hepatomegaly (online). Available at: https://pedclerk. bsd.uchicago.edu/page/hepatomegaly (accessed 11 February 2018).

Weledji, E. and Sinju, M. (2016). Delay in diagnosis of congenital anal stenosis. *Journal of Paediatric Surgery CASE REPORTS*, 5–8.

Wolf, A.D. and Lavine, J.E. (2000). Hepatomegaly in neonates and children. *Pediatrics in Review*, **21**: 303–10.

Further resources

Public Health England (2016/17). *Examination of the Testes. Newborn and Infant Physical Examination Programme Handbook.* London: PHE, pp. 20–1.

Stanford Medicine (2017). Newborn nursery: photo gallery (online) Available at: https://med.stanford.edu/newborns/professional-education/photo-gallery.html.

6E The skeletal examination

Sarah Paterson

Introduction

In this section we explore hip and foot problems in the newborn. Timely assessment of the hips by an expert is one of the public health key performance indicators in the newborn, and as such rates of achievement are recorded nationally.

Developmental dysplasia of the hip

Key points

- Developmental dysplasia of the hip is one of the most common orthopaedic conditions seen in childhood.
- If not detected in infancy it can lead to a lifetime of disability.
- Examination can be difficult in newborn babies, but recognition of those who may be at risk can significantly improve detection.

Introduction

Developmental dysplasia of the hip (DDH) describes a spectrum of abnormalities of the hip ranging from minor laxity to full dislocation. Recorded rates of DDH requiring treatment vary from 1–2 per 1000 babies born to 6–7 per 1000 (Jones, 1994; National Screening Committee, 2004). Intrauterine restriction of fetal movement in the latter stages of pregnancy is believed to be a major contributing factor in causing DDH, although genetic and hormonal factors may also play a part.

Current Public Health England newborn infant physical examination (NIPE) standards and NHS Quality Improvement Scotland best practice guidelines state that all neonates should have their hips examined as part of the NIPE or Scottish Routine Examination of the Newborn (SREN) within 72 hours of birth by a trained healthcare professional (NHS Quality Improvement Scotland, 2008; Public Health England, 2018). This examination is recommended to involve the use of Ortolani's and Barlow's stability tests along with observation and recognition of factors that may predispose the infant to DDH. If DDH is detected at this stage, it can be very effectively treated using a simple brace, which allows the infant to have full resolution of the condition in 97% of cases (Wilkinson and Wilkinson, 2010).

The NIPE and SREN are described as the primary examination. Identification of babies at risk at this stage allows timely referral to secondary screening programmes, which in turn will identify those infants who have a positive diagnosis of DDH, and subsequently allow implementation of effective conservative treatment.

If DDH is not detected at this examination or subsequent examination by the GP at 6–8 weeks of age, they will present 'late'. A late presentation of DDH is defined as being detected after age 12 weeks. In this situation it is unlikely that the infant will be able to be treated by conservative methods and will go on to require surgery, and often develop early onset osteoarthritis and a requirement for hip replacement. Up to 29% of hip replacements in adults aged less than 60 years are due to DDH (Furnes et al., 2001). There is considerable variation in published late presentation rates across the UK.

There are several factors that contribute to DDH not being detected in these first few weeks of life. Often those performing the examination have no or little experience, and there is no standardisation to teaching or examination. These factors lead to poor technique and lack of understanding of babies who may be at risk. As late presentations often occur at 18 months to 2 years of age, there is a long latent period after the newborn examination which makes feedback on accuracy of the original examination difficult

---

THINK POINT

Consider what other factors might make examination of a newborn infant's hips difficult.

The hip joint

The hip joint is a ball (femoral head) and socket (acetabulum) joint. The acetabulum should be deep enough to allow the femoral head to be well contained (Figure 6E.1). In the neonate the bone still has to ossify so it is cartilaginous in nature. If the femoral head does not sit properly in the acetabulum, it can become shallow. If the acetabulum is shallower than it should be, it can be described as DDH. The abnormality can vary in severity from a very minor irregularity to a very shallow hip, which allows the femoral head to move in and out (dislocate) of the acetabulum (Figure 6E.2). Due to the cartilaginous nature of the hip joint and the laxity of the surrounding tissues, this is rarely painful in the newborn.

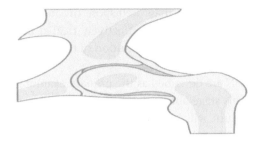

Figure 6E.1
Normal hip joint

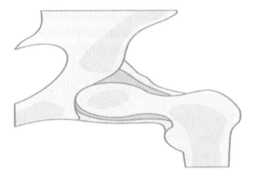

Figure 6E.2
Dysplastic hip joint

THINK POINT

- Consider what directions a hip joint should move in normally.
- What direction of movement is hip abduction and what direction of movement is hip adduction?

The cause of DDH is most probably multi-factorial; however, restriction of intrauterine movement (particularly hip abduction) during the last few weeks of pregnancy is thought to be a significant factor. The fetus is commonly vertex just before birth, with its left side towards the mother's spine. As the spine is less compliant, this can cause a reduction in abduction of the left hip. In an adducted position the femoral head will push out of the acetabulum, causing moulding of the cartilaginous surface and leading to poor congruency of the joint. DDH is more commonly seen in the left hip and this is believed to be the reason.

DDH is also more prevalent in bigger, overdue, long, first-born females, which can also be attributed to position *in utero*. What is difficult to determine is what we define as higher birth weight, length, etc. because this is most likely relative to the size of the mother.

Infants at risk

Due to the pathology of DDH there are certain factors that will predispose an infant to the condition and increase their risk. Recognition of these factors is vital to the successful screening of the newborn.

THINK POINT

Considering the pathology, can you identify any factors that may predispose an infant to DDH?

There are many traditional, well-documented risk factors predisposing babies to DDH, namely family history, breech presentation and oligohydramnios (Chan et al., 1997); however, between 40% and 75% of cases have no known risk factor (Wilkinson, 2011). It is therefore important to identify other signs that may indicate that there has been a restriction of movement *in utero*. The section on examination will help you to identify these.

Examination

Examination of a neonate's hips is not a simple tick box activity, whereby hips are definitively normal or abnormal. It should be a thorough examination that allows identification of factors that increase the risk of an infant having DDH. The infant should be settled, warm and comfortable. You should consider the order of your newborn examination, perhaps examining hips after auscultating the heart at the start of the examination. The infant must be partially undressed to allow full observation of position and the lie of the lower limbs. They should be on a flat, stable surface and cannot be effectively examined in a parent's arms. The nappy should be removed.

Observation

The infant should be observed at rest from top to toe for any signs of moulding:

- Start at the head, looking for any evidence of significant head preference, plagiocephaly, torticollis or significant moulding to the ears.
- Observe the infant's lying posture looking for any asymmetry, preferential lie to one side or apparent scoliosis
- Finally observe the feet looking for any evidence of a calcaneovalgus foot deformity (see section on feet below).

These are all signs of moulding or intrauterine restriction and put the infant at risk of DDH. As a primary examiner, it is important that you identify these features and ensure referral to a secondary screening programme.

Movement and skin creasing

Ensuring that your infant is settled, place your thumb web space over the infant's flexed knees. Remember that sudden movements or pushing hard on your infant will make them resist, thus making your examination more difficult.

- Gently flex the hips to 90° with knees flexed and in this position gently abduct both hips at the same time (Figure 6E.3).
- Normal range of motion in a newborn should allow the thigh to be abducted parallel to the cot mattress.
- Observe for any asymmetry in motion or loss of movement (Figure 6E.4).
- Observe for any asymmetry in groin or gluteal creases (deeper, extended line).

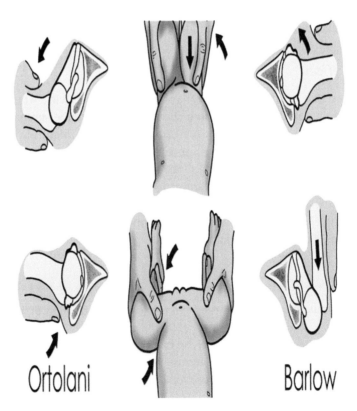

Figure 6E.3
Assessment of range of hip abduction

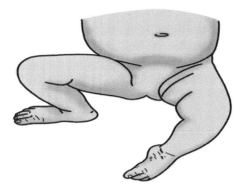

Figure 6E.4
Asymmetrical posture

- Due to the physiological flexion in a newborn infant, leg lengths can be difficult to assess at this stage. Also, at birth hips will sit more within the joint space than outwith, so there is often no obvious leg-length discrepancy even in a severely dysplastic hip. Leg-length discrepancy generally becomes increasingly obvious with age.

THINK POINT

Consider how the infant is lying: would you be concerned about the hips? Which hip and why?

Beware that some cases can be bilateral and asymmetry may not be such a significant feature however the infant will usually have a loss of abduction of the hips.

Stability tests

The two stability tests recognised as the standards for hip examination in a newborn are Ortolani's and Barlow's.

- Ortolani's test in 1937: described the hips held at 90° flexion and then a relocation jolt being felt during hip abduction in the unstable hip.
- Barlow's test in 1961: recognised that not all dysplastic hips dislocated, but subluxed or were lax in nature. He described testing one hip at a time while stabilising the pelvis. Then with the hip at 90° degrees gently pushing along the line of the femur to feel a posterior sliding movement.

In reality most examiners now use a combination of these manoeuvres. The NIPE practitioner may find that supervising clinicians use slightly different hand holds when examining hips. As stated before, neither of these manoeuvres is painful and should not in itself, cause the infant distress. Fingertip pressure is all that is required to successfully assess stability and hard pressure will result in distress to the infant, a feeling of nothing abnormal to the examiner and potential damage to the hip joint.

Therefore:

- Examine one hip at a time.
- With your left hand cradle the pelvis by scooping around the infant's right buttock. If you can, stabilise the right leg with your left thumb. Then with your right hand place your thumb web space over the infant's left flexed knee, with the infant's hip flexed to 90°, ensuring that your thumb is over the infant's inner thigh. Place the middle finger of your right hand on to the infant's left greater trochanter (Figure 6E.5).
- Apply gentle posterior pressure through your right hand, feeling for any posterior movement. A stable hip has a firm end feel, but a dysplastic hip can be felt to glide backwards and then forward again as the pressure is released.
- Maintaining the gentle posterior pressure and keeping your hand hold the same, gently abduct the infant's left hip. If the hip is unstable the femoral head can be felt to jump forward as it relocates into the acetabulum. This usually occurs in the first 10–15° of abduction.
- Repeat on the opposite hip.
- Soft tissue clicks are normal and of no clinical significance. It is important to identify this sensation as different to a re-entry jolt or clunk.

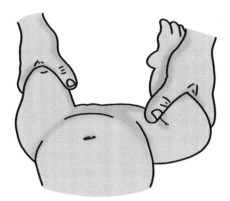

Figure 6E.5
Demonstration of hand position to assess for performing hip stability tests

In summary:

After examining a newborn infant's hips, as a primary examiner, you should consider making a referral to your local secondary screening programme if you encounter the following findings; however, you should also consult your local guidelines:

- Reduced hip abduction
- Features of moulding: ears, head, asymmetrical lie, calcaneovalgus feet
- Family history in first-degree relative (Public Health England, 2018)
- Breech presentation at or after 36 weeks of pregnancy (irrespective of presentation at delivery) (Public Health England, 2018)
- Extended breech presentation at delivery if this is earlier than 36 weeks. (Public Health England, 2018)
- Oligohydramnios
- Unstable or lax hips on clinical testing
- Uncertainty following hip examination.

Identification and early referral of the babies at risk of DDH allow urgent expert examination and ultrasound scans as appropriate, which is recommended by Public Health England to be within 2 and 6 weeks of life.

Treatment

The decision on whether an infant requires treatment for hip dysplasia is usually based on clinical and ultrasound findings after referral to a secondary screening programme. Treatment in this age group can successfully be achieved using a hip abduction orthosis – the most commonly used is the Pavlik harness. This will provide stability to the hips while the acetabulum re-models. It is generally well tolerated by the infant and can be extremely successful if used appropriately.

CLINICAL TIP

- Examination of hips in the newborn can be difficult and, as such, the NIPE practitioner should always refer to secondary screening if any suspicion of doubt occurs during clinical examination.
- An infant who is irritable or crying and kicking will always make examination more difficult, so the NIPE practitioner should take time to console or feed the infant before continuing to examine them.
- The NIPE practitioner should consider how they deliver the results of their findings to parents. Presenting information fully and concisely will help parents to understand and hopefully reassure them that the concerns are being dealt with appropriately and promptly.

Foot abnormalities in the newborn

Key points

- Clubfoot is the most common structural abnormality of the foot in the newborn.
- Identification of whether a foot abnormality is structural or positional in nature is extremely important because failure to do so can cause unnecessary appointments and parental anxiety.
- The aim of treatment in structural foot deformities is to achieve an adequate weight-bearing structure, but achievement of a 'normal' foot is not always possible.

Introduction

Babies can be born with a number of foot abnormalities that can be structural or positional in nature. These vary greatly in severity and subsequent long-term outcome. As the NIPE practitioner, it is important to be able to assess and identify these in order to ensure correct referral paths and that parents receive the correct advice. Sometimes foot abnormalities in babies can be related to other morbidities such as cardiac conditions, syndromes, chromosomal conditions and multi-joint abnormalities. It is therefore important to view the foot abnormality in context with other findings during the NIPE, and seek senior review if required because the infant may need further clinical or genetic testing.

> **THINK POINT**
>
> Can you identify any syndromes that may have clubfoot as a clinical sign.

This section gives you a guide on how to assess a newborn foot, the types of foot abnormality that you might encounter, and some basics around treatment and outcomes.

Examination of the newborn foot

The infant should be at least partially undressed with their feet and legs exposed. They should be on a flat stable surface.

> **THINK POINT**
>
> Consider what movements should occur at the ankle and foot and what a normal degree of movement for a newborn is.

Observation

The infant should be observed at rest and ideally during movement. You should consider:

- What position the foot is in at rest – downwards (plantarflexion), inwards (inversion), upwards (dorsiflexion), outwards (eversion) or a combination of these
- Does the infant's foot have a straight lateral border?
- Does this change as the infant wriggles and kicks, and by how much?
- Does the infant have five toes?
- Does the foot look shorter than the other foot (if one foot affected)?
- Does the great toe look shorter than the other toes?
- Are there any significant creases in the foot more than normal fine lines?

Movement and feel

- Steady the infant's leg around the knee or upper shin and with your other hand grasp around the toes. Never hold around the heel (Figure 6E.6).
- Attempt to move the foot to the neutral position to see how far the foot corrects. This should be a gentle movement and never be forceful. If a foot points down and in, try correcting by taking the foot out and up. Conversely if the foot points up and out, try taking the foot down and in.
- Feel for any abnormal bony prominences on the lateral and medial sides of the foot.
- Feel the heel pad; this should feel firm like pressing on your forehead, but may represent a structural abnormality if it feels like pushing on the tip of your nose or your cheek (Figure 6E.6).

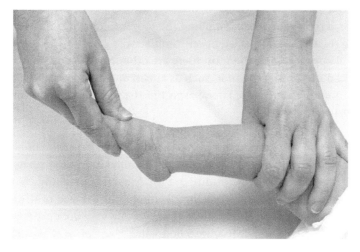

Figure 6E.6
Demonstration of hand position to assess movement in a baby's foot

Evertor stimulation

- While holding around the knee or upper shin try 'tickling' the outside lateral border of the foot to see if this stimulates the muscles to correct the foot posture either fully or partially.

Clubfoot or congenital talipes equinovarus

Clubfoot is a complex structural abnormality of the foot. The foot points downwards (equinus) and inwards (varus). The incidence varies worldwide and is reported between 1 and 4 per 1000 live births, (Carroll, 2011); however, in Europe the incidence is thought to be 1.2 per 1000 (Siapkara and Duncan, 2007) The cause is still generally unknown, although for the most part it is a developmental condition that occurs *in utero*. This means that, with the introduction of the 20-week fetal anomaly scan being available to all expectant mothers, clubfoot is in most cases detected antenatally. There is a familial link with clubfoot, which it is often seen running in families but not necessarily in a first-degree relative. The familial occurrence is believed to be multifactorial in nature. Approximately 50% of cases are bilateral and it occurs twice as frequently in boys as girls.

Clubfoot is a multijoint, multidirectional deformity and will not resolve spontaneously. It is important for you as the NIPE practitioner to identify this from a positional equinovarus foot posture. There are some classic features that can help with this process:

1 Creasing: in a structural clubfoot there will be a significant posterior crease just above the heel and also creasing in the medial arch of the foot (Figure 6E.7).
2 General mobility: in a structural clubfoot the foot will be unable to be fully corrected with gentle movement.
3 Evertor activity: the muscles pulling the foot into dorsiflexion and eversion will be sluggish or non-existent on stimulation.
4 General appearance of the foot: there are other features that may be apparent when examining the foot, such as apparent shortening of the great toe, bony prominences on the lateral aspect of the foot and a soft empty feel to the heel pad.

Clubfoot is now most commonly treated using Ponseti's method of correction. This method of treatment utilises a series of manipulations and plaster casts to correct each element of the deformity in turn. Most require a surgical release of the Achilles tendon and then bracing overnight till the age of 4 or 5 years. Although the results of this treatment are generally very good, it is important to remember that the feet will always be treated clubfeet, and as such display small features that have the potential to cause some, albeit minor, influences to normal activities of daily life. The NIPE practitioner should always be aware

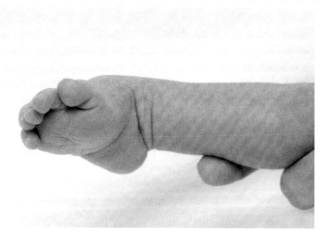

Figure 6E.7
Posterior and medial creasing observed in clubfoot

that, when the clubfoot has been diagnosed antenatally, many parents will have received counselling. This means that they will be well informed on treatment and outcomes and can at times appear quite relaxed about the diagnosis.

> ## THINK POINT
>
> - Consider the emotions a parent may be experiencing if their infant's clubfoot was not diagnosed antenatally.
> - How might you address this?

When clubfoot has not been diagnosed antenatally parents often ask: 'Will my infant walk?' When clubfoot occurs in isolation, it is expected that they will achieve their developmental milestones as normal and parents should be reassured of this. However, when other pathologies are present, this is not always true and your answer should be somewhat guarded, suggesting that opinion should be sought from specialist services to ascertain the answer. Some centres may recommend senior medical review of any infant born with clubfoot but the NIPE practitioner should refer to their local guidelines for this.

Referral should be made to your nearest paediatric orthopaedic specialist offering Ponseti's technique. No interim stretching should be given because this can be detrimental to the clubfoot.

Positional equinovarus foot

As the name suggests the foot is held in a similar position to the clubfoot but there will be no obvious signs of creasing (other than normal fine lines) and the foot will easily be fully corrected. There should also be evidence of at least partial correction on performing evertor stimulation. If this is the case, the foot can be deemed to be positional in nature and is most likely caused by malposition *in utero*. This is a common feature, which self-resolves in nature over the first few weeks of life; as such there is no evidence to support intervention (Hart, 2009). NIPE practitioners should avoid giving this type of foot a formal diagnosis because the term 'talipes' or 'positional malalignment of the foot' is widely used but is poorly defined on the internet, and therefore not differentiated from the far more significant deformities such as clubfoot. This can cause undue stress to parents.

Metatarsus adductus

A foot that displays metatarsus adductus will have an entirely normal hind-foot, but will be adducted from the mid-portion at the metatarsals, resulting in a curve to the lateral border. It can on initial observation resemble a club-foot, but on closer inspection the signs of hindfoot involvement (posterior creasing and softening to the heel pad) will be absent (Figure 6E.8). Metatar-sus adductus is poorly observed in newborns and, as such, there is little recorded about the incidence. However, it is believed generally to be self-resolving in nature over the first few months of life (Hossain and Davis, 2017). The NIPE practitioner should assess the foot for medial creasing and flexibility if they suspect this may be the diagnosis. In this scenario a referral should be made to the nearest paediatric orthopaedic specialist for further review. Occasionally the use of plaster casting and bracing is required. (Hossain and Davis, 2017).

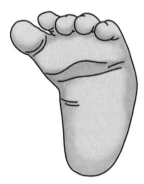

Figure 6E.8
Plantar view of metatarsus adductus foot – note the medial crease and splay of the great toe and second toe

Calcaneovalgus foot posture

In a calcaneovalgus foot, the foot is markedly dorsiflexed and everted (Figure 6E.9). It occurs in approximately 6 in 1000 live births (Chotigavanichaya et al.,

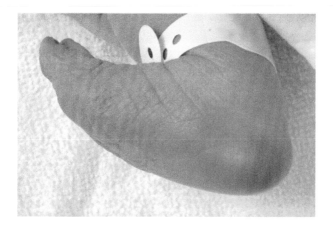

Figure 6E.9
Medial view of calcaneovalgus foot – note extreme dorsiflexion of the hindfoot with
normal creasing

2012). Although the problem is positional in nature, plantarflexion is often
limited to only the neutral position. On first observation the heel often looks
abnormal but, as the foot is inverted and plantarflexed, the heel will automati-
cally drop into the normal position. The foot posture can look quite alarming
to parents, but it is in fact self-resolving and again there is no evidence to
support any intervention.

However, there is an association between calcaneovalgus foot posture and
DDH in the contralateral side. If a calcaneovalgus foot posture is observed the
NIPE practitioner should consider referring the infant for secondary hip
screening.

Congenital vertical talus

Congenital vertical talus (CVT) is an extremely rare structural abnormality
occurring in around 1 in 10,000 live birth (Jacobsen and Crawford, 1983)
(Figure 6E.10). As many as 50% of cases occur as part of a syndrome or have
related pathologies (Watson, 2014). CVT is sometime mistaken for clubfoot
during antenatal scanning. You might find some clinical supervisors refer to
this as a rocker-bottom foot but the NIPE practitioner is encouraged to use the
medical terminology.

As with clubfoot, CVT is a multidirectional deformity and will not resolve
spontaneously. It can on first observation resemble a calcaneovalgus foot
posture, so the NIPE practitioner must take care on examination to identify the
difference. There are some classic features that can help with this process:

1   Creasing: unlike the calcaneovalgus foot the hindfoot in a CVT is in fact in
    equinus. As a result of this there will be a deep posterior crease and empty/
    soft heel pad on palpation, much the same as in a clubfoot.

2   General mobility: the foot will be stiffer and unable to be corrected to the mid-line.

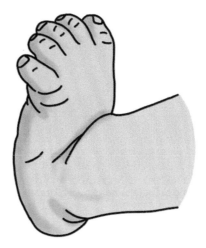

Figure 6E.10
Congenital vertical talus foot – note posterior creasing and hindfoot in equinus

CVT is now most commonly treated using the reverse Ponseti's technique (Dobbs et al., 2007). This also utilises a series of manipulations and plaster casts to reduce the talus, followed by a surgical release of the Achilles tendon and concurrent pinning of the talonavicular joint. This is usually followed by a period of splinting, but there is great variation in this between clinicians.

As with clubfoot, the results are generally good; however, given the common association with other abnormalities, the NIPE practitioner should be guarded in their predictions of outcomes to parents at the time of the NIPE.

CLINICAL TIP

• The NIPE practitioner should always ensure that they gather a full antenatal history from the parents to ascertain whether any abnormalities have been previously detected.

• It is important that the NIPE practitioner considers the findings of a foot abnormality ,along with any other positive findings of the newborn examination (particularly cardiac). A senior review can be helpful to ascertain whether these factors are related.

• NIPE practitioners should familiarise themselves with their local referral procedures/treatment centres.

• NIPE practitioners should remember that there is no clinical indication for them as a primary examiner to implement any treatment.

THINK POINT

Consider how you might approach discussions over diagnosis and treatment for an infant who has not been diagnosed antenatally, but you are concerned has a structural foot abnormality.

Polydactyly and syndactyly and absence of toes

Polydactyly (duplication of toes) and syndactyly (webbing of toes) are relatively common anomalies at birth. They can occur in isolation or be associated with other conditions. Syndactyly frequently requires no treatment, so the NIPE practitioner should simply reassure parents of this. Polydactyly will usually result in simple removal surgically, but this is often not performed until at least the age of 1 year. Occasionally there can be a more complex problem with the underlying skeletal structure, which can result in a less satisfactory outcome in the longer term. An infant found to have polydactyly should be referred non-urgently to your nearest local paediatric orthopaedic service for further review.

Absence of toes can often occur as a result of amniotic band syndrome in which the full development of a limb is affected *in utero*. There can be a more complex underlying structural abnormality as a result of this, and it is often seen in association with an altered foot posture. Often a tight band can be felt further up the limb (frequently in the calf region). A careful examination of the lower limbs should be conducted by the NIPE practitioner, with consideration given to the previous foot examination section. If an infant is found to have absence of toes they should be referred to your nearest local paediatric orthopaedic service for further review.

References

Carroll, N.C. (2011). Clubfoot in the twentieth century: where we were and where we may be going in the twenty-first century. *Journal of Pediatric Orthopaedics B*, **21**: 1–6.

Chan, A., McCaul, K.A., Cundy, P.J., Haan, E.A. and Byron-Scott, R. (1997). Perinatal risk factors for developmental dysplasia of the hip. *Archives of Disease in Childhood – Fetal and Neonatal Edition*, **76**(2): F94–100.

Chotigavanichaya, C., Leurmsumran, P., Eamsobhana, P., Sanpakit, S. and Kaewpornsawan, K. (2012). The incidence of common orthopaedic problems in newborn at Siriraj Hospital. *Journal of the Medical Association of Thailand*, **95**(9): 54–61.

Dobbs, M.B., Purcell, D.B., Nunley, R. and Morecuende, J.A. (2007). Early results of a new method of treatment for idiopathic congenital vertical talus. Surgical technique. *Journal of Bone and Joint Surgery of America*, **89**(Suppl 2, Pt 1): 111–21.

Furnes, O., Lie, S.A., Espehaug, B., Vollset, S.E., Engesaeter, L.B., Havelin, L.I. (2001). Hip disease and the prognosis of total hip replacements. A review of 53698 primary total hip replacements reported to the Norwegian Arthroplasty Register 1987–99. *Journal of Bone and Joint Surgery of Britain*, **83**: 579–86.

Hart, D. (2009). *Physiotherapy Management of Positional Talipes Equinovarus*. Evidence Note 01. London: Chartered Society of Physiotherapy.

Hossain, M. and Davis, N. (2017). Evidence-based Treatment for Metatarsus Adductus. In: Alshryda, S., Huntley, J. and Banaszkiewicz, P. (eds), *Paediatric Orthopaedics*. Champagne, IL: Springer.

Jacobsen, S.T. and Crawford, A.H. (1983). Congenital vertical talus. *Journal of Pediatric Orthopedics*, **3**: 306–10.

Jones, D.A. Principles of screening and congenital dislocation of the hip. *Annals of the Royal College of Surgeons of England*, **76**: 245–50.

National Screening Committee (2004). Child Health subgroup report: Dysplasia of the hip, 2004.Available at: https://legacyscreening.phe.org.uk/hipdislocation.

NHS Quality Improvement Scotland (2008). Best practice statement: Routine examination of the newborn, 2008. Available at www.healthcareimprovement scotland.org/previous_resources/best_practice_statement/examination_of_the_ newborn.aspx (accessed April 2018).

Public Health England (2018). NHS Newborn and infant physical examination (NIPE) screening programme. Available at: www.gov.uk/government/ publications/newborn-and-infant-physical-examination-screening-standards (accessed April 2018).

Siapkara, A. and Duncan, R. (2007). Congenital talipes equinovarus. A review of current management. *Journal of Bone and Joint Surgery of Britain*, **89**: 995–1000.

Watson, L. (2014). Congenital vertical talus. *APCP Journal*, **5**(2): 24–8.

Wilkinson, A.G. and Wilkinson, S. (2010). Neonatal hip dysplasia: A new perspective. *NeoReviews*, **11**(7): e349–62.

Wilkinson, S. (2011). Physiotherapist-led neonatal hip screening programme: A ten-year review. *APCP Journal*, **2**(3): 27–44.

Further resources

Barlow, T. (1966). Early diagnosis and treatment of congenital dislocation of the hip in the newborn. *Proceedings of the Royal Society of Medicine*, **59**: 1103–6.

Ortolani, M. (1976). Congenital hip dysplasia in the light of early and very early diagnosis. *Clinical and Orthopaedics and Related Research*, **119**: 6–10.

Examination of the skin

Natalie Anders and Alison Cooke

As a student or qualified midwife you will be the first professional to come into contact with the newborn at delivery. This is a perfect opportunity to assess the naked baby and fully appreciate the appearance of the newborn's skin. The next opportunity for a professional to observe the baby naked may be during the newborn infant physical examination (NIPE) which will be carried out by you as a qualified NIPE practitioner or another NIPE-trained professional. This group of professionals also includes neonatal nurses. Neonatal nurses will often examine babies of less than 37 weeks' gestation who have spent time on a neonatal unit. It is important to be aware of your own trust guidance on which babies you are qualified to examine. Any practitioner caring for mothers and babies on the neo-natal unit or the postnatal ward will be the parents' first point of reference for any questions that they may have about their baby's skin.

This chapter will assist you to understand the anatomy of the skin structure and enable you to recognise some of the common and rarer conditions that you might highlight during a NIPE.

THINK POINT

Consider what skin conditions you have previously encountered during your examinations of babies in your care.

Physiology of the skin

The integumentary system, consisting of the skin and accessory structures such as the hair, nails, sweat and oil glands, is the largest organ in the human body in relation to surface area and weight (Moini, 2016). The fundamental functions of the skin are a barrier against infection, thermoregulation, prevention of insensible fluid loss and mechanical protection (Fimiani et al., 2012). There are three main layers to the skin (Figure 6F.1), consisting of the outer layer or epidermis, the middle layer or dermis and the underlying layer of subcutaneous fat (Gordon and Lomax, 2015).

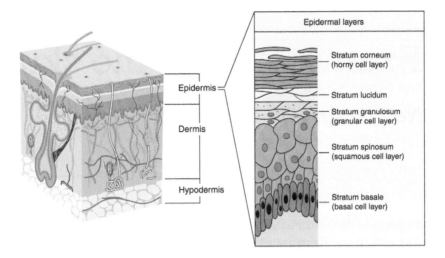

Figure 6F.1
Skin structure

Although the newborn skin is structurally similar to that of an adult, it is more immature, which makes it more permeable and fragile (Witt, 2016). For example, the stratum corneum is 30% thinner and the overall epidermis is 20% thinner in babies compared with adults (Stamatas et al., 2010). The ratio of body surface to body weight is higher for babies than for adults, increasing permeability (Nikolovski et al., 2008), and a baby's skin remains in a state of transition for up to 2 years of life (Nikolovski et al., 2008; Fluhr et al., 2011; Stamatas et al., 2011). At birth the fetus is covered in vernix caseosa, a thick white material composed of exfoliated skin cells, proteins and sebaceous gland secretions, which thickens in the third trimester and serves as a barrier to protect the skin (Witt, 2016). A fine downy hair called lanugo will also cover the fetus from around 20 weeks' gestation until it starts to disappear at around 40 weeks (Witt, 2016).

Assessment of the skin

A systematic assessment of the skin can assist the practitioner in identifying the presence of infection or disease (petechiae or vesicles), organ dysfunction (pallor, cyanosis and jaundice), nutritional status and gestational age. The assessment should include the inspection and palpation of the skin, identifying colour, tone, texture, turgor, integrity and birthmarks.

> ## THINK POINT
>
> Before examining the baby, what information could you find in the maternal antenatal and intrapartum history that may lead you to look for certain skin concerns?

Before examining the skin the maternal history should be reviewed for potential or diagnosed problems. Previous history that could affect the skin includes: sexually transmitted infections, immune status, rhesus disease or any haemolytic disease, the gestation at delivery, position at delivery and length of labour, method of delivery and any antenatal concerns diagnosed by ultrasound scan. Each of these could manifest as a change in the appearance of the newborn skin.

THINK POINT

What is the best environment in which to examine the newborn's skin?

To achieve an accurate assessment of the skin, it is essential to examine the baby in the most appropriate environment to support this. This requires appropriate natural lighting, correct room temperature and no distractions. It is important that the baby can be fully examined without clothing to identify any normal or abnormal findings (Gleason and Juul, 2012). The temperature needs to be optimal to avoid vascular changes to the skin appearance and to maintain the baby's temperature. The light source should be natural to ensure that any pigment changes can be accurately assessed and the skin is not tinted by unnatural light (Dinulos, 2015).

THINK POINT

Consider your trust's guidance; what steps should you take to report and refer a skin finding?

Although skin findings such as non-infectious rashes or spots are quite common in the newborn period, and often transient and benign, they need to be fully visualised to distinguish them from serious skin infections. These findings then need further follow-up depending on what the diagnosis is. It is safer to seek reassurance or a second opinion from a more experienced practitioner, be that another neonatal nurse, midwife or paediatrician. The parents can be fully updated on the findings once the practitioners involved have a diagnosis because they will often need reassurance about the health of their baby. All assessment findings should be documented in the baby's notes to educate all caregivers about the baby's situation (Nursing and Midwifery Council, 2015). This also provides the opportunity to highlight any lesions that were identified at birth or have subsequently developed. Accurate documentation will provide other practitioners involved in the baby's care with a contemporaneous history of the baby's skin condition.

This chapter now examines some common skin conditions that a NIPE practitioner might highlight during the examination.

Normal newborn lesions

Milia

Milia are smooth cysts 1–2 mm in size, white in colour, filled with keratin (Figure 6F.2). Milia are found mainly on the newborn face (Asrani and Wanner, 2011). They do not require intervention and should disappear within the first few weeks of life. If there are any further concerns from the parents about the milia, such as a change in appearance, then they should be advised to seek a further review from their general practitioner.

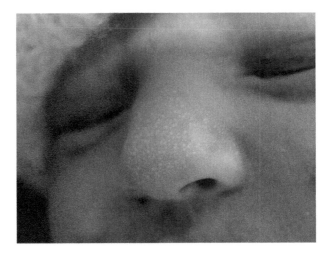

Figure 6F.2
Milia (image courtesy of ADHB Neonatal Dermatology)

Erythema toxicum neonatorum

Erythema toxicum neonatorum is one of the most common benign skin conditions (Figure 6F.3), occurring in at least half of term newborns, although less prevalent in preterm babies (Wright and Cohen, 2012). This condition usually commences at about 24 hours of age and spontaneously resolves by around day 5; however, new lesions can develop up to day 10 (Gloster et al., 2015). Lesions will present as small white pustules or papules on an erythematous (red) base, typically starting on the face and spreading to the trunk and limbs (Phung et al., 2017). The palms and soles of the feet are usually spared and it is common to find worsening rash in moist areas such as creases of the groin, joints and neck. If this rash is identified, the practitioner can examine the baby's skin and palpate to see if it blanches. By pressing lightly on the spotty rash, it should become pale and fade. The practitioner should ensure that there are no other accompanying symptoms which could indicate an infection as the cause of the rash, such as lethargy, temperature instability or poor feeding. If the rash is blanching and there are no other concerns about the baby the

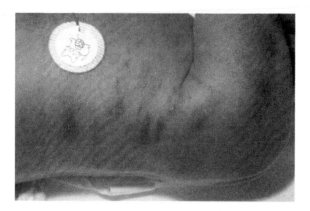

Figure 6F.3
Erythema toxicum neonatorum (image courtesy of ADHB Neonatal Dermatology)

practitioner can advise the parents that the rash should spontaneously resolve within 2 weeks and that they should resist picking or squeezing the spots. However, if it worsens or the baby becomes unwell, then the practitioner should advise the parents to seek further support from their general practitioner.

Neonatal acne

Neonatal acne (Figure 6F.4) is more common in males than females due to the production or presence of hormonal androgens, increasing sebum excretion and stimulation of the sebaceous glands (Al-Mutairi, 2016). It is also known to be caused by an inflammatory response to an overgrowth of normal neonatal skin flora (Al-Mutairi, 2016). The lesions occur from birth to 1 month of age,

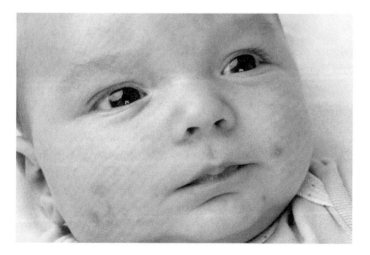

Figure 6F.4
Neonatal acne

primarily on the face, and can be open or closed comedones, papules and pustules (Al-Mutairi, 2016). Advice should be given to the parents to seek further support if the acne persists beyond this time frame because virilisation should be excluded.

Sucking blister

This is a blister without surrounding inflammation caused by vigorous intrauterine sucking reflex (Baston and Durward, 2017). The blister or erosion (if it has burst) can be found on the limbs, hands or fingers (Figure 6F.5). It can also be seen on the lips from sucking when feeding. These blisters should resolve within a few days; however, if there are an increased number evident or the blisters are inflamed, then a diagnosis should be sought. If the baby is discharged at this point the parents should be advised to see their general practitioner.

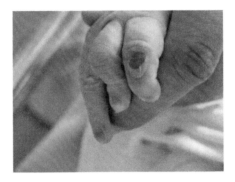

Figure 6F.5
Sucking blister (image courtesy of ADHB Neonatal Dermatology)

Miliaria

Miliaria (Figure 6F.6) is also known as heat rash and is caused by the keratinous obstruction of the sweat ducts (McCollum and Friedlander, 2010). Miliaria rubra, also known as prickly heat, can be caused by friction from clothing or overdressing. Miliaria presents as clusters of papules or vesicles surrounded by an erythema (McCollum and Friedlander, 2010). Miliaria crystallina is more superficial, presenting as thin-walled vesicles with no erythema, and mainly found in skinfolds (McCollum and Friedlander, 2010). Parents should be advised that the rash should resolve within a few days; however, they can help to resolve the current rash by reducing heat and humidity in the rooms that the baby occupies, placing the baby in the shade, avoiding synthetic fibres by opting for natural fibre clothing that is loose fitting, and using cool baths to help to soothe the baby if they seem uncomfortable. Lotions should be avoided unless recommended by the pharmacist or general practitioner.

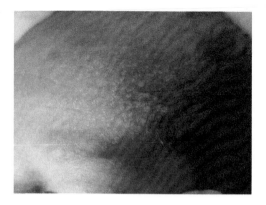

Figure 6F.6
Miliaria (image courtesy of ADHB Neonatal Dermatology)

Seborrhoeic dermatitis

Seborrhoeic dermatitis is a greasy scaly rash, usually confined to the scalp area [image (a) in Table 6F.1], but may also be seen on the forehead and eyebrow area. It is commonly termed 'cradle cap'. This can be caused by an overactivity of the sebaceous gland, resulting from circulating maternal hormones (Trotter, 2010). The scaly yellow crusts on the scalp are easily identifiable and the parents should be advised that it will spontaneously resolve within a week to a few months without treatment. No medical intervention is required unless the scalp bleeds, swells or spreads across the face and body.

Transient neonatal pustulosis

Transient neonatal pustulosis (Figure 6F.7) is characterised by vesiculopustules on a non-erythematous base and is more common in the African-American

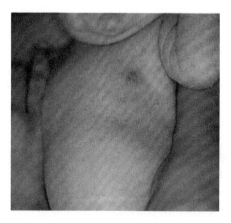

Figure 6F.7
Transient neonatal pustulosis (image courtesy of Dr Thomas Hubiche, Fréjus, France [Boralevi and Taïeb, 2011])

population (Phung et al., 2017). The lesions can be present at birth or appear soon after anywhere on the body. Once the delicate pustules rupture they leave behind hyperpigmented macules, which will resolve over a few weeks (Phung et al., 2017). No laboratory tests are required for this condition because it should resolve without treatment; the parents should not need any further medical intervention. If midwives are unsure of a diagnosis at birth, they should seek a review from the paediatrician to confirm the diagnosis. The parents can be informed that it is unlikely after the first day or two for any further blisters to develop. If further blisters do develop, the baby may need a further review by a medical professional.

Colour

Acrocyanosis

Acrocyanosis is peripheral cyanosis and is a normal finding in neonates up to several hours after birth, causing the hands and feet to appear blue in colour (Whitaker et al., 2015). Peripheral cyanosis is caused by vasomotor instability and can appear worse with cold stress. It should be differentiated from central cyanosis which is characterised by a blue colouring to the skin and mucous membranes and could indicate underlying hypoxaemia (see Chapter 6B) (Breinholt, 2012). Visualising cyanosis can be ambiguous and difficult in newborns with pigmented skin; however, the mucous membranes can give an indication if examined. To differentiate between a bruise and cyanosis, depression of a bruise should not change its appearance; however, an area of cyanosis will blanch (Flannery, 2013). If in any doubt as to the cause of the cyanosis, the baby will need a further review by a paediatrician.

Plethora

Plethora is a red skin coloration that can be an indication of excessive red blood cells (polycythaemia). Polycythaemia is classified as a haematocrit level above 0.65l/l and can be caused by delayed cord clamping or milking of the umbilical cord, maternal diabetes mellitus or twin-to-twin transfusion (Fimiani et al., 2012). This can be a normal finding in newborns that will settle; however, these newborns could be more at risk of developing jaundice when the excess red blood cells break down. The NIPE practitioner should be fully aware of neonatal jaundice and its management.

In this scenario the practitioner should take a full maternal history, looking for evidence of any haemolytic disease or whether there have been any previous babies diagnosed with jaundice in the family. The practitioner should also consider any history of birth trauma or increased infection risk. The baby's current situation should be noted, identifying the feeding history, an accurate assessment of input and output, and presenting time of jaundice considering

CASE STUDY 1

You are carrying out the NIPE of a term baby, who is 50 hours old and exclusively breastfeeding. The mother reports that she initially had some difficulty establishing breastfeeding. However, during the last breastfeed, she had some support from the infant feeding team and the baby effectively latched on to her breast and fed well. On examination of the skin you find that the baby appears to be jaundiced. What history should you consider and what are your actions?

whether the jaundice could be pathological or physiological. Once all of the factors are assessed, a plan should be put in place to carry out a diagnostic test. A transcutaneous bilirubinometer can be used and further blood samples can be obtained including serum bilirubin, full blood count and direct antiglobulin test. Feeding support should be offered to the mother and baby to ensure that poor feeding is not contributing further to the jaundice levels. If the diagnostic test confirms jaundice, then treatment in the form of phototherapy should be offered. This treatment should be followed up by further monitoring of the bilirubin levels on a phototherapy treatment graph appropriate for the baby's gestation (National Institute for Health and Care Excellence [NICE], 2014). All management and care should follow your trust's guideline.

Jaundice

Neonatal jaundice, demonstrated by the yellowing of the skin, sclera and mucous membranes, is caused by an imbalance in the production and excretion of bilirubin (Ricci and Kyle, 2009). *In utero* unconjugated bilirubin passes the placenta and is conjugated by the maternal liver and excreted (Ricci and Kyle, 2009). Bilirubin levels should be normal at the time of birth (Ricci and Kyle, 2009).

Red blood cells are broken down to produce haem and globin. Biliverdin is a byproduct of this, which is converted into bilirubin, a yellow pigment, that causes jaundice (Gordon and Lomax, 2015). The bilirubin is attached to albumin and transported to the liver to become conjugated and water soluble, so it can then be excreted in the stool or urine (Gordon and Lomax, 2015). In the gut the bacteria converts bilirubin to urobilinogen to allow reabsorption from the gut, and then to be excreted by the kidneys in the urine (Gordon and Lomax, 2015). This function in newborns is immature because *in utero* the process relies on the placenta, leading to an increased risk of jaundice. The risk is also increased by newborns having a higher turnover of red blood cells and fewer bacteria in the gut. This leads to the conjugated bilirubin becoming deconjugated and there is increased enterohepatic circulation as a result (Gordon and Lomax, 2015).

Physiological jaundice, a normal finding, peaks by day 3–5 and has a total bilirubin rise of <5 mg/dl per day (Choudhury, 2018). Pathological jaundice, an abnormal finding, is when jaundice occurs within the first 24 hours of life and has a bilirubin rise of <0.2 mg/dl per hour (Choudhury, 2018).

If jaundice is suspected and the baby is over 24 hours old, a transcutaneous bilirubinometer should be used to assess the severity within a 6-hour period (NICE, 2010). If this demonstrates a reading of 250 μmol/l, then a serum bilirubin measurement should be taken and plotted on the appropriate gestation graph to determine whether treatment is required (NICE, 2010). If jaundice is suspected at less than 24 hours old, a serum bilirubin measurement should be taken and the infant reviewed by a paediatrician to assess for other contributing factors.

Harlequin colour change

This phenomenon [image (b) in Table 6F.1] usually presents around age 3–4 days and is defined by a colour difference on the right and left sides of the body. The affected side will be the side the baby is lying on and will be erythematous to the midline, with the face of the baby remaining pale in colour (Boralevi and Taïeb, 2011). This phenomenon is considered to have no pathological significance; it may be caused by immature hypothalamic centres and poor control of peripheral vascular tone (Boralevi and Taïeb, 2011). If this phenomenon occurs the practitioner should seek a medical review to confirm a diagnosis. Providing that the examination of the newborn is normal no further action is required. The parents should be educated that, if the colour change continues for over 4 weeks, then cardiac lesions that cause poor perfusion should be ruled out. The baby is given this length of time to allow the immature hypothalamic centres to mature, potentially ruling this out as a cause. Although the newborn examination aims to identify any cardiac abnormalities through auscultation and saturation monitoring, it is a screening rather than a diagnostic test, so some abnormalities could potentially be missed. Ongoing review can continue to assess the health of the baby and allow the practitioner to make appropriate referrals.

Collodion baby/ichthyosis

The skin of a collodion baby [image (c) in Table 6F.1] at birth has the appearance of a yellow, shiny and tight film covering the skin. It is more common in babies born prematurely (<37 weeks' gestation). Further examination of the baby does not usually provide any abnormal findings but the baby's movement may appear restricted. The membrane or 'film' may not completely cover the baby and it may be localised to specific areas. It may peel away, but then it may reappear and this process may continue over several weeks. Usually the membrane gradually disappears within 1–4 weeks; however, for some babies this can take up to 3 months. In most cases, once the membrane has shed, the baby remains with an erythrodermic or lamellar ichthyosis as seen in image (d) of Table 6F.1 (O'Toole and Kelsell, 2011).

The condition is associated with an impaired skin barrier function which may mean that the baby will suffer from increased transepidermal heat and water loss, so practitioners should be observant of hypothermia and dehydration (Buyse et al., 1993). Due to the symptoms of this condition and also the baby's high ratio of skin surface to body weight resulting in increased permeability, the baby may be susceptible to rapid systemic toxicity if topical agents are used on the skin surface (O'Toole and Kelsell, 2011). Practitioners should therefore use any skin treatments with caution.

As the condition has a propensity to prematurity, these babies will usually be cared for in the neonatal unit. Care after this will depend on the baby's condition. Most babies will be discharged within the first 6 weeks after birth. A care management plan will be provided by the paediatric team. In those units that do not have consultant paediatric dermatologists, the baby should promptly be referred to the doctor on call for the maternity unit, who can then review the condition and make an appropriate outpatient appointment or referral.

Infectious skin disorders

Herpes simplex virus

Antenatally herpes simplex virus (HSV) can be transmitted through contact with open genital lesions at delivery, or postnatally through contact with active lesions in caregivers or visitors. In newborns the lesions present as clusters of blisters that can burst and crust over (Charlton, 2015).

Charlton (2015) characterises infections as:

1 Disseminated, involving multiple organs, with or without central nervous system (CNS) involvement
2 CNS involvement, encephalitis, with or without skin/eye or mouth involvement
3 Localised to the skin, mouth or eyes.

Antenatal treatment can be commenced prophylactically according to the trust's policy if lesions are active at the time of delivery. The mode of delivery would be by planned caesarean section to reduce the risk of transmission. If a baby is diagnosed with HSV, then an antiviral treatment should be commenced immediately while waiting for the blood tests to confirm the presence of the infection. Dependent on the classification of the baby's disease, admission to the newborn intensive care unit may be necessary.

THINK POINT

Which factors should you be aware of that can increase the risk of maternal-to-newborn transmission of HSV?

Contributory factors may include prolonged rupture of the membranes, integrity of the membranes, mode of delivery, and whether the maternal infection is primary or recurrent. Primary infections or those that occur closer to delivery are associated with a higher risk than secondary infections or those that occur in early pregnancy.

THINK POINT

If a mother discloses to you that she has HSV, what would your action plan be for care?

In this scenario if the disclosure is made before delivery, the practitioner would recommend and arrange prophylactic treatment for the mother and consider alternative delivery modes. If the disclosure was made post-delivery the practitioner should observe the baby for signs and symptoms of infection and refer to the medical team, who will consider the appropriateness of further tests or antibiotic treatment for the baby. If the baby is preterm or has broken skin, and there are active maternal lesions after a vaginal delivery, a course of treatment may be necessary.

Candida

Candida rash can be a common finding in newborns. The rubbing of delicate skin with prolonged exposure to stool or urine in a moist environment can create an overgrowth of the yeast *Candida* species (Rudolf et al., 2011). This can also be caused after a change in gut flora following a course of antibiotics

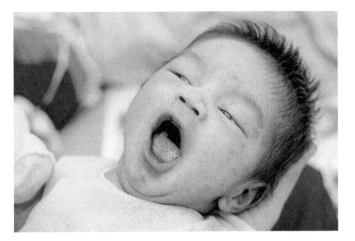

Figure 6F.8
Oral candida infection

(Rudolf et al., 2011). The rash will be very bright red and more common in the skinfolds of the groin, with some vesicles and pustules around the rash (Rudolf et al., 2011). Many parents may find that, despite home treatments or barrier creams, the rash will remain for 2–3 days. Nappy rash can be accompanied by oral thrush, which will be presented as white curds on the buccal mucosa (Figure 6F.8). If this rash occurs, the parents need to seek medical advice because they may need an antifungal treatment to resolve the nappy and oral rash. Parents may also find that the newborn may be uninterested in feeding if the mouth is sore. It is important to keep the baby hydrated. All utensils and bottles should be properly washed and sterilised because poor hygiene can cause oral thrush. If thrush is found during the NIPE then, as a practitioner, you will need to arrange the appropriate treatment.

Staphylococcal scalded skin syndrome

This skin disorder presents as generalised erythema with a pyrexia, followed by formation of large blisters that can cause partial-thickness skin loss if they rupture as shown in image (e) of Table 6F.1 (Sieber et al., 2012). This results in fluid loss, hypothermia, electrolyte imbalance and a secondary infection (Sieber et al., 2012). These babies would need immediate medical review to determine the extent of the rash, with antibiotic coverage and possible fluid management.

Pigmented lesions

Mongolian blue spot

This blue–grey blemish has a bruise-like presentation. Although the most common site to find the blemish is just above the buttocks, it is important to be aware that this mark could be found anywhere on the body [image (f) of Table 6F.1].

THINK POINT

Why is it important to accurately document this birthmark?

Due to the nature of the blemishes appearing like bruises, it is important to document their location and size at birth to alert any other professionals of their site and size. This is to distinguish these marks from non-accidental injury.

Café-au-lait spots

Café-au-lait spots are brown patches [image (g) of Table 6F.1] that become darker with time, representing areas of increased keratinocytes and melanin

(Gordon and Lomax, 2015). It should be noted that multiple spots can be associated with neurofibromatosis (Gordon and Lomax, 2015). The spots themselves are benign and do not cause any problems; however, they should be documented accurately in the baby's medical notes. Size, location and number should be documented. More than six spots of at least 5 mm in diameter in pre-pubertal children is one of the major diagnostic criteria of neurofibromatosis (Gordon and Lomax, 2015). The parents should be educated about the longer-term implications and given advice to seek further medical intervention should the number of spots increase as the baby grows.

Congenital melanocytic naevus

This is a mole-like mark on the skin or large pigmented lesion. The surface can be pigmented in shades of brown or blue and covered with hair. Small naevi (small brown birthmarks) require no further intervention or follow-up. Large naevi or large, hairy, deeply pigmented lesions require urgent referral to the consultant paediatric dermatologist to review potential treatment or surgical options. The medical team should be alerted to these birthmarks and accurate documentation should be maintained. In those units that do not have consultant paediatric dermatologists; the baby should be promptly referred to the doctor on call for the maternity unit, who can then review the lesion and make an appropriate outpatient appointment or referral.

Vascular lesions

Naevus simplex (stork bite)

Dilated capillaries cause a flat, pink discoloration of the skin around the eyelids, the bridge of the nose or the nape of the neck (McKinney et al., 2013) (Figure 6F.9). The discoloration can become more prominent when the baby

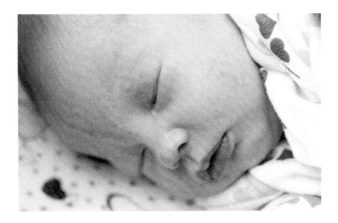

Figure 6F.9
Naevus simplex

cries but will resolve without intervention by around 2 years of age. There is no further follow-up or treatment required other than reassuring the parents that the discoloration will fade and spontaneously resolve in time. The size and location should be documented in the baby's notes.

Port wine naevus

A port wine naevus is a flat pink to dark-red mark which can present anywhere on the body and varies in size (Figure 6F.10). This will not blanch with pressure and can be removed only with laser treatment (McKinney et al., 2013). This mark can be associated with certain syndromes such as Klippel–Trenaunay syndrome, Parkes–Weber syndrome, Servelle–Martorell syndrome, proteus syndrome and Bannayan–Riley–Ruvalcaba syndrome. A non-urgent referral should be made to the consultant paediatric dermatologist and accurate documentation of the size and location should occur. In those units that do not have a consultant paediatric dermatologist, the baby should promptly be referred to the doctor on call for the maternity unit, who can then review the lesion and make an appropriate outpatient appointment or referral.

Infantile haemangioma (strawberry haemangioma)

This is a dark-red, uneven mark, which consists of enlarged capillaries in the outer layer of the skin (McKinney et al., 2013). The haemangioma is normally located on the head [image (h) of Table 6F.1] and will peak in size at around 6 months of age, with regression over several years until it disappears (McKinney et al., 2013). Treatment will be required only if the haemangioma invades the

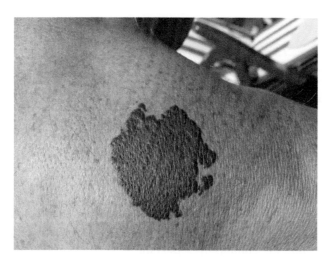

Figure 6F.10
Port wine naevus

eye area or becomes infected. The size and location should be documented in the baby's notes. Parents should be informed to seek further medical intervention depending on how the haemangioma grows, and to monitor for signs of infection.

Cavernous haemangioma

Cavernous haemangioma is similar to the infantile haemangioma; however, it is more vascular and involves endothelial cells, the dermis and subcutaneous tissues (Witt, 2016). The haemangioma will be soft to touch with poorly defined borders, and the overlying skin will be blue/red in colour (Witt, 2016). The haemangioma will increase in size over the first year after birth before it spontaneously involutes [images (i, j) in Table 6F.1]. If the haemangioma impedes the function of vital organs it can be shrunk with corticosteroid therapy.

Cavernous haemangioma is associated with the Kasabach–Merritt and Klippel–Trenaunay–Weber syndromes. The Kasabach–Merritt syndrome is characterised by thrombocytopenia, anaemia and impaired clotting, possibly caused by a lymphatic malformation with underlying venous connections (Witt, 2016). The Klippel-Trenaunay–Weber syndrome is caused by malformation of the blood vessels and excess blood flow, resulting in hypertrophy of the bone and other organs, with a vascular naevus (Witt, 2016). The medical team should review this before discharge, and a referral to the consultant paediatric dermatologist should be made for follow-up. Accurate documentation enables follow-up appointments to determine the extent of the growth. In those units that do not have a consultant paediatric dermatologist, the baby should promptly be referred to the doctor on call for the maternity unit, who can then review the lesion and make an appropriate outpatient appointment or referral.

THINK POINT

Consider, when examining the skin, why it is important as the NIPE practitioner that you review the birth history.

Trauma lesions

Forceps and Ventouse-assisted delivery

Most commonly bruising or lacerations to the temples or cheeks can be seen from a forceps injury. Ventouse-assisted delivery may commonly incur bruising to the scalp, but less commonly a laceration, although this is possible. It is important to assess the depth of any laceration and offer parents advice about healing because these are usually self-limiting injuries. However, more rarely there can be damage to the nerves causing a palsy, fractures or haemorrhages. These should be immediately assessed to put in place the correct follow-up plans and treatment. The midwife at the delivery will complete a risk management form for all birth injuries. This ensures that practice can be monitored to ensure that maternity professionals are providing safe and evidence-based practice. Physiotherapy referrals will be made for the baby if this is appropriate. For most facial palsy this will be as an outpatient appointment. If the face has lacerations, depending on the extent of these, then a referral to the plastics team may be warranted.

Newborn skin care

During the NIPE examination parents often ask the practitioner about caring for their baby's skin, so it is important that practitioners are aware of the current evidence base. Care of the newborn skin commences in the delivery room once the newborn has been born. Parents should be encouraged to provide skin-to-skin time with their baby to allow maternal–offspring exchanges of microbiota. This will allow the baby's microbiome to develop (Mueller et al., 2015) to enhance immune (Fung et al., 2012) and metabolic (Cox et al., 2014) health.

With regard to day-to-day care for the skin, historically parents and healthcare workers have believed that water alone is best to care for the newborn skin (Lavender et al., 2009). However, a systematic review found that there was no significant difference between the use of specific baby wash-and-wipe products compared with water alone in relation to skin surface hydration, skin pH, skin assessment scores or erythema (Cooke et al., 2018). This evidence provides parents with a choice of how to care for their baby's skin supported by robust evidence.

The review also found that, in those babies who have a genetic predisposition to the development of atopic eczema, there is strong evidence to indicate the use of daily, full-body emollient application (Cooke et al., 2018). However, in healthy term babies who have dry skin, the review found that using commonly recommended oils on the skin, such as olive oil and sunflower oil, adversely affected the development of the skin barrier and that these oils should not be recommended (Cooke et al., 2018). Evidence suggests that dry skin is normal for newborn term babies and will usually resolve within 3–4 weeks without any treatment (Cooke et al., 2016). For preterm babies cared for on a neonatal unit, including those without a genetic predisposition to atopic eczema, emollients may be recommended in trust policies for newborn dry skin (Lund and Durand, 2015). There is consequently a difference in guidance for dry skin care between preterm and term babies. This is driven by a desire to reduce the prevalence of skin infection in preterm babies that can adversely affect the prognosis of an already vulnerable baby (Darmstadt et al., 2004).

Use of adhesives should be minimal because the removal of these can strip the epidermis, tear the skin and cause sensitisation (Lund and Durand, 2015).

Table 6F.1 Skin disorders and conditions

(a) Seborrhoeic dermatitis

(Image courtesy of Gelmetti and Grimalt [2011]; © 2011 Blackwell Publishing Ltd)

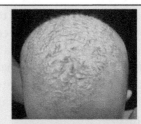

(b) Harlequin colour change

(Image courtesy of Boralevi and Taïeb [2011]; © 2011 Blackwell Publishing Ltd)

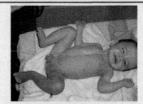

(c) Collodion baby

(Image courtesy of O'Toole and Kelsell [2011]; © 2011 Blackwell Publishing Ltd)

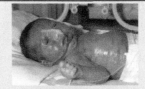

(d) Lamellar ichthyosis

(Image courtesy of O'Toole and Kelsell [2011]; © 2011 Blackwell Publishing Ltd)

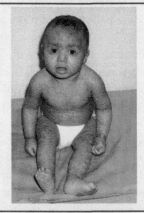

(e) Staphylococcal scaled skin syndrome

(Image courtesy of Ott and Hoeger [2011]; © 2011 Blackwell Publishing Ltd)

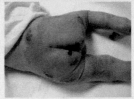

Table 6F.1 Continued

(f) Mongolian blue spot

(Image courtesy of Newton-Bishop [2011];
© 2011 Blackwell Publishing Ltd)

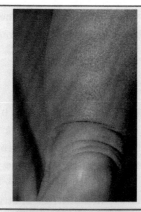

(g) Café-au-lait spots

(Image courtesy of Newton-Bishop [2011];
© 2011 Blackwell Publishing Ltd)

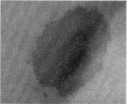

(h) Strawberry haemangioma

(Image courtesy of Bruckner and Frieden
[2011]; © 2011 Blackwell Publishing Ltd)

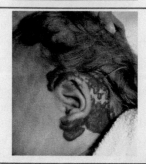

(i, j) Haemangioma associated with
Kasabach–Merritt syndrome: (i) image of a
2-month-old infant with Kasabach–Merritt
syndrome. (j) The same child at age 7 years
after treatment with a course of prednisone
and a Coban wrap.

(Courtesy of Bruckner and Frieden [2011];
© 2011 Blackwell Publishing Ltd)

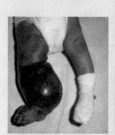 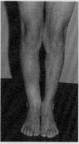

The cord should be allowed to dry naturally. If redness around the umbilical stump occurs and appears to be worsening or appears tender to touch with a smelly odour or discharge, further medical intervention should be sought to have the area assessed for infection and to receive treatment if required.

Conclusion

This chapter has provided you with information on the anatomy of the skin structure and some of the common and rarer skin conditions that you might highlight during a NIPE. There will always be opportunities for skin conditions that you may not have seen before to come to your attention in practice. It is important to remain within your own sphere of knowledge and refer to the most appropriate clinician when in any doubt.

References

Al-Mutairi, N. (2016). Neonatal acne controversies versus pityrosporum folliculitis. In: Oranje, A., Al-Mutairi, N. and Shwayder, T. (eds), *Practical Pediatric Dermatology Controversies in Diagnosis and Treatment*. Geneva: Springer International Publishing.

Asrani, F. and Wanner, M. (2011). Care and maintenance of normal skin. In: Schalock, P., Hsu, J. and Arndt, K. (eds), *Lippincott's Primary Care Dermatology*. Philadelphia, PA: Wolters Kluwer Health.

Baston, H. and Durward, H. (2017). *Examination of The Newborn: A Practical Guide*, 3rd edn. London: Routledge.

Boralevi, F. and Taïeb, A. (2011). Common transient neonatal dermatoses. In: Irvine, A., Hoeger, P. and Yan, A. (eds), *Harper's Textbook of Pediatric Dermatology*, 3rd edn. Oxford: Blackwell Publishing, pp. 6.1–12.

Breinholt, J. (2012). Cardiac disorders. In: Cloherty, J., Eichenwald, E., Hansen, A. and Stark, A. (eds), *Manual of Neonatal Care*. Philadelphia, PA: Wolters Kluwer Health/Lippincott Williams & Wilkins.

Buyse, L., Graves, C., Marks, R., Wijeyesekera, K., Alfaham, M. and Finlay, A. (1993). Collodion baby dehydration: the danger of high transepidermal water loss. *British Journal of Dermatology*, **129**: 86–8.

Charlton, F. (2015). The skin. In: Khong, T. and Malcomson, R. (eds), *Keeling's Fetal and Neonatal Pathology*, 5th edn. Geneva: Springer.

Choudhury, S. (2018). *Pediatric Surgery*. Singapore: Springer.

Cooke, A., Cork, M., Victor, S., Campbell, M., Danby, S., Chittock, J. and Lavender, T. (2016). Olive oil, sunflower oil or no oil for baby dry skin or massage: a pilot, assessor-blinded, randomized controlled trial (the Oil in Baby SkincaRE [OBSeRvE] study). *Acta Dermato-Venereologica*, **96**: 323–30.

Cooke, A., Bedwell, C., Campbell, M., McGowan, L., Ersser, S. and Lavender, T. (2018). Skin care for healthy babies at term: A systematic review of the evidence. *Midwifery*, **56**: 29–43.

Cox, L., Yamanishi, S., Sohn, J., Alekseyenko, A., Leung, J., Cho, I. et al. (2014). Altering the intestinal microbiota during a critical development window has lasting metabolic consequences. *Cell*, **158**: 705–21.

Darmstadt, G., Badrawi, N., Law, P., Ahmed, S., Bashir, M., Iskander, I. et al. (2004). Topically applied sunflower seed oil prevents invasive bacterial infections in preterm infants in Egypt. *Pediatric Infectious Disease Journal*, **23**: 719–25.

Dinulos, J. (2015). Dermatologic conditions. In: MacDonald, M. and Seshia, M. (eds), *Avery's Neonatology*, 7th edn. Philadelphia, PA: Wolters Kluwer.

Fimiani, M., Bilenchi, R., Mandato, F., Mei, S., Nami, N. and Strangi, R. (2012). Neonatal skin disorders. In: Buonocore, G., Bracci, R. and Weindling, A. (eds), *Neonatology*. Milan: Springer.

Flannery, V. (2013). Assessment of the normal newborn. In: Murray, S., McKinney, E., Holub, K. and Jones, R. (eds), *Foundations of Maternal–Newborn and Women's Health Nursing*, 6th edn. Maryland Heights, MO: Elsevier Health Sciences.

Fluhr, J., Darlenski, R., Lachmann, N., Baudouin, C., Msika, P., DeBelilovsky, C. and Hachem, J. (2011). Infant epidermal skin physiology: adaptation after birth. *British Journal of Dermatology*, **166**: 483–90.

Fung, I., Garrett, J.P., Shahane, A. and Kwan, M. (2012). Do bugs control our fate? The influence of the microbiome on autoimmunity. *Current Allergy and Asthma Reports*, **12**: 511–19.

Gelmetti, C. and Grimalt, R. (2011). Infantile seborrhoeic dermatitis. In: Irvine, A., Hoeger, P. and Yan, A. (eds), *Harper's Textbook of Pediatric Dermatology*, 3rd edn. Oxford: Blackwell Publishing, pp. 35.1–8.

Gleason, C. and Juul, S. (2012). *Avery's Diseases of the Newborn*, 9th edn. Philadelphia, PA: Elsevier Saunders.

Gloster, H., Mistur, R. and Gebauer, L. (2015). *Absolute Dermatology Review*. London: Springer.

Gordon, M. and Lomax, A. (2015). The neonatal skin: examination of the jaundiced newborn and gestational age assessment. In: Lomax, A. (ed.), *Examination of the Newborn*, 2nd edn. Chichester: Wiley Blackwell.

Lavender, T., Bedwell, C., Tsekiri-O'Brien, E., Hart, A., Turner, M. and Cork, M. (2009). A qualitative study exploring women's and health professionals' views of newborn bathing practices. *Evidence Based Midwifery*, **7**: 112–21.

Lund, C. and Durand, D. (2015). Skin and skin care. In: Merenstein, G. and Gardner, S. (eds), *Merenstein and Gardner's Handbook of Neonatal Intensive Care*, 8th edn. St Louis, MO: Mosby Elsevier.

McCollum, A. and Friedlander, S. (2010). Dermatologic emergencies. In: Crain, E. and Gershel, J. (eds), *Clinical Manual of Emergency Pediatrics for PDA*, 5th edn. Cambridge: Cambridge University Press.

McKinney, E., James, S., Murray, S., Nelson, K. and Ashwill, J. (2013). *Maternal–Child Nursing*, 4th edn. Maryland Heights, MO: Elsevier Saunders.

Moini, J. (2016). *Anatomy and Physiology for Health Professionals*, 2nd edn. Burlington, MA: Jones & Bartlett Learning.

Mueller, N., Bakacs, E., Combellick, J., Grigoryan, Z. and Dominguez-Bello, M. (2015). The infant microbiome development: mom matters. *Trends in Molecular Medicine*, **21**: 109–17.

National Institute for Health and Care Excellence (NICE) (2010). *Neonatal Jaundice. Clinical Guideline no. 98*. London: NICE.

National Institute for Health and Care Excellence (2014). *Postnatal Care. NICE Clinical Guideline 37:* London: NICE.

Nikolovski, J., Stamatas, G., Kollias, N. and Wiegand, B. (2008). Barrier function and water-holding and transport properties of infant stratum corneum are different from adult and continue to develop through the first year of life. *Journal of Investigative Dermatology*, **128**: 1728–36.

Nursing and Midwifery Council (NMC) (2015). *The Code: Professional standards of practice and behaviour for nurses and midwives*. London: NMC.

O'Toole, E. and Kelsell, D. (2011). Collodion baby. In: Irvine, A., Hoeger, P. and Yan, A. (eds), *Harper's Textbook of Pediatric Dermatology*, 3rd edn. Oxford: Blackwell Publishing.

Phung, T., Wright, T., Pourciau, C. and Smoller, B. (2017). *Pediatric Dermatopathology*. London: Springer.

Ricci, S. and Kyle, T. (2009). *Maternity and Pediatric Nursing*, 2nd edn. London: Wolters Kluwer.

Rudolf, M., Lee, T. and Levene, M. (2011). *Paediatrics and Child Health*, 3rd edn. Chichester: Wiley-Blackwell.

Sieber, D., Abood, G. and Gamelle, R. (2012). Necrotizing and exfoliative diseases of the skin. In: Jeschke, M., Kamolz, L., Sjöberg, F. and Wolf, S. (eds), *Handbook of Burns*. Vienna: Springer.

Stamatas, G., Nikolovski, J., Luedtke, M., Kollias, N. and Wiegand, B. (2010). Infant skin microstructure assessed in vivo differs from adult skin in organization and at the cellular level. *Pediatric Dermatology*, **27**: 125–31.

Stamatas, G., Nikolovski, J., Mack, M. and Kollias, N. (2011). Infant skin physiology and development during the first years of life: a review of recent findings based on in vivo studies. *International Journal of Cosmetic Science*, **33**: 17–24.

Trotter, S. (2010). Neonatal skincare. In: Holmes, D. and Lumsden, H. (eds), *Care of the Newborn by Ten Teachers*. London: CRC Press.

Witt, C. (2016). Skin assessment. In: Tappero, E. and Honeyfield, M. (eds), *Physical Assessment of the Newborn*, 5th edn New York: Singer Publishing Co.

Whitaker, K., Eberle, P. and Trujillo, L. (2015). *Comprehensive Perinatal and Pediatric Respiratory Care*, 4th edn. Boston, MA: Cengage Learning.

Wright, D. and Cohen, B. (2012). Common newborn dermatoses. In: *Avery's Diseases of the Newborn*, 9th edn. Philadelphia, PA: Elsevier Saunders.

7 Congenital abnormalities

Joanne Cookson

The aim of this chapter is to consider some congenital abnormalities that may be identified during the newborn infant physical examination (NIPE). The role of the practitioner in the diagnosis and the subsequent management is explored. Also key considerations with regard to the identification of congenital abnormalities before, during and after the NIPE are discussed.

Congenital abnormalities continue to be the leading cause of infant mortality (Sinha et al., 2017), as well as a key contributor to childhood and adult morbidity (Vrijheid et al., 2000). It is important that, as a NIPE practitioner, you feel well prepared to consider the potential diagnosis of a congenital abnormality when signs and symptoms are identified as part of the NIPE screening process.

Definition

Congenital anomalies affect around 2% of newborn babies (EUROCAT, 2018). A congenital abnormality is often referred to as a birth defect, congenital malformation or congenital disorder. Such abnormalities have a variety of causes, including pregnancy or birth complications, genetic malformations, viral infections or drug exposure *in utero* (Lalani, 2017). However, in many cases, a congenital anomaly may have no known cause. Congenital anomalies can be defined as structural or functional anomalies that occur during intrauterine life. With advances in antenatal screening, many of these congenital anomalies are identified before birth, either during an ultrasound examination or following non-invasive screening for fetal aneuploidy, and the subsequent diagnostic tests such as chorionic villous sampling (CVS) or amniocentesis. Such invasive testing is usually offered to women after a high-risk screening test result, a family history of chromosome abnormality, other genetic disease or an abnormal ultrasound scan. It is important to consider that such antenatal screening does not identify all congenital abnormalities and the NIPE practitioner should be aware of this. Some congenital anomalies will be detected only at birth or sometimes may be detected only as the child develops (World Health Organization [WHO], 2016).

Current issues

Worldwide the impact of congenital abnormalities continues to be a significant contributor to mortality and morbidity issues. It is estimated that 303,000 newborns die within 4 weeks of birth every year due to congenital anomalies (WHO, 2016). Where longer-term disability develops as a consequence of the congenital abnormality, this has a significant impact not only on the individual but also on their support network of family, as well as impacting on healthcare systems and society.

Causes and risk factors

Although approximately 50% of all congenital anomalies cannot be linked to a specific cause, there are some known genetic, environmental, and other causes or risk factors.

Genetic factors are responsible for some congenital abnormalities. This might be because of damaging changes within genes, known as mutations, or because the fetus has too much or too little genetic material.

THINK POINT

Consider other socioeconomic and demographic factors that may increase the possibility of a congenital abnormality.

Low income

There is a higher incidence of congenital abnormalities in resource-constrained families and countries (Vrijheid et al., 2000). It has been estimated that about 94% of severe congenital abnormalities occur in low-income families (WHO, 2016). This increase may be explained by a lack of access to appropriate nutrition which is known to reduce the risk of congenital abnormalities, such as the reduction in spina bifida associated with preconceptual folic acid supplements. Such factors can increase the likelihood of abnormal prenatal development. Women from lower socioeconomic families are also less likely to access antenatal screening.

Maternal age

Advanced maternal age increases the risk factor for certain chromosomal abnormalities, including Down's syndrome. NIPE practitioners should be aware of the changing demographic population accessing our maternity services. The Office for National Statistics (2016) has confirmed that, for the first time ever, women over 40 are the only age group with a growing pregnancy rate in the UK.

Consanguinity

Consanguinity has been linked to increases in the prevalence of rare genetic babies born in consanguineous relationships, which nearly doubles the risk for neonatal and childhood death, intellectual disability and some other anomalies (WHO, 2016). The risk in consanguineous relationships is that there is a greater chance that both parents may carry a defective gene for a recessive condition. If the child inherits a defective gene from each parent, he or she will be affected with the genetic disease, which, in some conditions, results in a congenital anomaly. It has been suggested that, of children born from consanguineous relationships, up to 53% can present with congenital anomalies (Chitkara, 2016).

THINK POINT

Consider why a pregnancy that has occurred from a consanguineous relationship might be at a higher risk of a congenital abnormality?

Environmental factors

Maternal exposure to certain pesticides and other chemicals, as well as noxious substances, increases the risk of having a newborn with a congenital abnormality (Sadler, 2015).

Infections

As alluded to in Chapter 6, maternal infections such as syphilis and rubella can cause congenital abnormalities. These issues remain a concern in many developing countries (WHO, 2016). A more recent cause of congenital abnormality is due to *in utero* exposure to the Zika virus. This has led to many newborns being born with significant microcephaly alongside other congenital abnormalities. At present there have been no cases identified in the UK, but practitioners undertaking the NIPE should be aware if women have visited at-risk countries during their pregnancy.

Maternal nutritional status

Pregnant women are advised to take extra folate supplementation; insufficient intake increases the risk of having an infant born with a neural tube defect. Excessive levels of vitamin A may affect the normal development of the fetus and should be limited; pregnant women may not always receive this important dietary advice.

Before the NIPE

It is imperative before completing the NIPE that a comprehensive assessment of the maternal notes is undertaken (Public Health England, 2018) (please refer to Chapter 5 for more details as to why this is so important). With regard to congenital abnormalities, it will help the NIPE practitioner identify if there are any positive antenatal screening results or diagnostic tests that have not been communicated within the multidisciplinary team (MDT), or any family history or socioeconomic considerations that may increase the chance of a child being born with a specific congenital abnormality. The practitioner may be alerted to the possibility of an abnormality just by reading the maternal notes.

During the NIPE: communication issues

In the event that a congenital abnormality is detected on the NIPE that has not been diagnosed antenatally, it is essential for the NIPE practitioner to be able to communicate the findings to the parents (see Chapter 3 on communication). Senior medical input should be sought to assist in this process; families require someone to provide an explanation of the diagnosis, and this should be given by a practitioner who has sufficient knowledge and experience to be able to give an honest and accurate account of what can be expected and the subsequent management.

The NIPE practitioner should very much be part of the team that communicates with the parents. The significance of potentially breaking bad news should never be underestimated. It is important for careful consideration to be given before the conversation begins. If a congenital abnormality is suspected, the news needs to be imparted in a sensitive manner.

The parents may not have any insight into any potential problems either immediate or in the future. An emotional response is to be expected because the parents' expectations of the perfect infant may be shattered. Parents may display conflicting emotions, such as grief and anger, and may initially reject the infant or the diagnosis. The NIPE practitioner should be prepared to manage such an emotional response. Ensure that parents are aware that the significance of the news is appreciated; remain calm with the ability to respond to questions. Before the discussion, the practitioner should have an awareness of the referral process and agencies that will be involved in the management of the infant and the family.

Parents should be given time to absorb the information. It may be necessary to revisit parents while they remain in hospital as more questions arise. In such situations there is a need to avoid multiple consultations with different healthcare professionals, although if a genetic cause is suspected the infant may need to be examined by a clinical genetics consultant. Wherever possible, parents should be seen by the same consultant paediatrician or advanced neonatal practitioner (ANNP) until the infant has been discharged from hospital.

Although congenital anomalies may be the result of one or more genetic, infectious, nutritional or environmental factors, it is often difficult to identify the exact causes. This makes the communication in this situation extremely difficult because parents will often want to know why this has occurred to their child.

Please refer to Chapter 3 for further information on communication issues during the NIPE.

THINK POINT

Consider the breaking of significant news where English is not the parents' first language. What strategies would you consider to ensure that the message is delivered in an effective way?

Genetic causes of congenital malformations

Genetic causes are reported to be responsible for 15–25% of congenital malformations observed during the first year of life.

A brief summary of some of the more common genetic conditions associated with congenital abnormalities is given below to highlight some of the signs and symptoms that may present at birth, as well as outlining some of the associated short- and long-term consequences. Some genetic conditions can present with easily recognisable signs, for example Down's syndrome (trisomy 21), whereas others can be diagnosed only by an expert and require specific testing to confirm the diagnosis. It is important to note that some of these conditions are very rare.

Down's syndrome

This is the most common chromosomal birth abnormality affecting 1 in 800–1000 births. Rather than having the usual number of 46 chromosomes, a person with Down's syndrome has 47 (there are 3 copies of chromosome 21 instead of the usual 2; hence you will often hear it called trisomy 21). This extra chromosome is usually caused by a mistake during the development of eggs or sperm, which results in the fertilised egg having 3 copies of chromosome 21. The risk of having an infant with trisomy 21 increases with maternal age, with women aged over 40 years having a risk of more than 1 in 100 (Loane et al., 2013).

Down's syndrome is characterised by a number of typical dysmorphic features such as a flattened bridge of the nose and epicanthic folds. The irises may have pale flecks within them known as Brushfield's spots. There may also by some degree of hypotonia, often characterised by a protruding tongue. The NIPE practitioner may notice that the head circumference is on the small side with a degree of brachycephaly. One of the most common features of Down's syndrome often cited is the single palmar crease. It is important to be aware that this feature is present in 5% of the normal population, so it is not diagnostic.

Many cases of Down's syndrome are identified through antenatal screening. Those women identified to be at increased risk are offered an amniocentesis or chorionic CVS and, in the advent of a positive diagnosis, can opt for a therapeutic termination of the pregnancy. Practitioners undertaking the NIPE should be prepared for approximately 30% of cases not being identified before birth (Down Syndrome Medical Interest Group – see www.dsmig.org.uk). This is mainly due to women declining antenatal screening.

> ## THINK POINT
>
> Sarah is 42 years old and has just given birth to her first child, Ellie. You have been asked to complete the NIPE; as you start your examination you notice some familial traits that are indicative of Down's syndrome. Sarah is married to Tom who is also present during the examination. Consider an appropriate management plan for Ellie and her parents.

If Down's syndrome is suspected by the practitioner completing the NIPE, there is a need to request a review by a paediatrician or an ANP. The NIPE practitioner needs to assess whether there is evidence of any cardiac, gastrointestinal or respiratory problems because these are more prevalent in neonates with Down's syndrome. It is estimated that 40% of infants with Down's syndrome will have an identifiable congenital heart defect (Ranweiler, 2009). Any related feeding issues should also be assessed because this may also pose a problem that may need resolving. A consultant paediatrician will need to discuss testing to confirm the diagnosis with the parents. An urgent genetic test should be requested to confirm trisomy 21. The suspected diagnosis should be shared with the parents so that they can give informed consent for the genetic testing.

Edwards' syndrome

Edwards' syndrome is the second most common chromosomal abnormality affecting 1 in 3000–5000 births. It is caused by the presence of an extra copy of chromosome 18. As with trisomy 21 and trisomy 13, most cases are diagnosed antenatally after screening or an ultrasound scan. Newborn babies with trisomy 18 will usually be small for gestational dates, and can present with a small abnormally shaped head, low-set ears, micrognathia, and heart and kidney abnormalities. Characteristic features of trisomy 18 are tightly clenched fists with overlapping little fingers and rockerbottom feet with prominent heels; these are often signs that are highlighted during antenatal ultrasound scans. The syndrome is incompatible with life and most infants will die within the first year. Urgent genetic testing should be requested to confirm trisomy 18. Survivors will have severe developmental delay.

Patau's syndrome

Patau's syndrome is very rare and has an incidence of around 1 in 5000–8000 births. It is caused by an extra copy of chromosome 13 and is often referred to as trisomy 13. It has a similar mechanism of origin as trisomy 21 and there is also an increased risk with advanced maternal age. Trisomy 13 is often detected during pregnancy through antenatal screening or by ultrasound scan. The malformations associated with trisomy 13 can be severe and this can be shocking for the parents. Sometimes the front of the brain does not develop properly, leading to a condition known as holoprosencephaly. This can result in severe bilateral cleft lip and palate; the eyes may be very close together or in a single eye socket and the nose may not form properly. Extra fingers and toes are a common occurrence. In some cases the abdominal wall does not develop properly, leading to an exomphalos developing. There is a high chance of a cardiac abnormality, with a cardiac defect identified in up to 80% of all cases. Trisomy 13 is incompatible with life with the most infants dying in their first year of life. Those children who survive will have severe developmental delay. Urgent genetic testing should be requested to confirm trisomy 13.

Turner's syndrome

Turner's syndrome affects only girls. It is caused by complete or partial loss of one X chromosome in female infants. It has an occurrence rate of 1 in 2000 (Turner Syndrome Support Society – see https://tss.org.uk). Although Turner's syndrome is often detected prenatally due to oedema detected on an ultrasound scan, it is not always apparent at birth and many girls are not diagnosed until childhood or adolescence. The features that may be present at birth include a short webbed neck with loose skin, low hairline and intrauterine growth restriction (IUGR). Oedematous hands and feet are often present (David et al., 2017). Some babies with Turner's syndrome will have cardiac and renal abnormalities. Infants develop a normal level of intelligence. The main features of Turner's syndrome are short stature and failure to enter puberty. Females with Turner's syndrome are almost always infertile due to ovarian failure (Oktay et al., 2016).

Early diagnosis enables growth hormone treatment to be started at an appropriate age, and age-appropriate puberty induction with hormone therapy can be planned. Unfortunately, less than 20% of girls are diagnosed before they are 12, so they do not receive the early diagnosis required to ensure the opportunity for life-changing therapies (Bondy, 2007).

DiGeorge's syndrome

DiGeorge's syndrome has an incidence of 1 in 4000 births. It is often referred to as a 22q11 deletion because cause is a missing part of the DNA from one parent (Rennie, 2012). NIPE practitioners should consider this diagnosis where a cleft palate or congenital heart disease is diagnosed, these being common features of the condition. NIPE practitioners should ensure that they adhere to the Royal College of Paediatrics and Child Health guidelines (RCPCH, 2015) on palate examination and inspect under direct vision with a torch and a tongue depressor to completely exclude a cleft palate being present. Often small cleft palates at the back of the oral cavity can potentially be undiagnosed unless this recommendation is adhered to.

Noonan's syndrome

Noonan Syndrome has an incidence of between 1 in 1000–2500 births. It is characterised at birth by unusual facial features. Children with Noonan Syndrome will often have short stature, webbed neck and have malformations of the bones and rib cage that leads to an unusual shaped chest with widely spaced and low set nipples. NIPE practitioners suspecting Noonan Syndrome should be aware that these children are at an increased risk of congenital heart defects (Romano et al., 2010).

Beckwith–Wiedemann syndrome

Beckwith–Wiedemann syndrome (BWS) is a very rare condition associated with overgrowth, with an incidence of approximately 1 in 15,000 live births. The genetic causes of BWS are complex. The condition is often not identified until birth, when identifying features may be noticed (Zammit et al., 2017). Features associated with BWS are macroglossia, abdominal wall defects, high birth weight and neonatal hypoglycaemia. Urological problems are also commonly associated with the condition, with renal abnormalities being a common issue.

Early recognition is essential to ensure life-saving interventions. Where the syndrome is suspected, blood glucose levels should be checked to rule out the development of hypoglycaemia. If macroglossia is present, the airway should be assessed for patency and relevant steps taken to ensure that the airway is kept open if a problem is identified. Assistance with feeding may also be required for the same reason.

Some children with BWS are at risk of a type of kidney cancer called Wilms' tumour, so it is important that they are examined by a clinical geneticist who can order genetic testing.

Prader–Willi syndrome

This syndrome is a rare disorder. Prevalence is estimated to be between 1 in 10,000 and 1 in 1:30,000 births. The genetics of Prader–Willi syndrome (PWS) is complex. PWS is not always identified at birth; neonates with this syndrome can present with a low birth weight. There is often hypotonia which develops prenatally, and can lead to reduced tone in the fetus with subsequent delivery via caesarean section being more common (Abdilla et al., 2017). This lack of tone means that babies are often described as floppy and will often have feeding difficulties that the parents will need support to resolve.

Facial features associated with the syndrome include a thin upper lip and mouth turned down at the corners and a narrow nasal bridge; the palpebral fissures are almond shaped (Abdilla et al., 2017). These facial features may not be recognised at birth and can become more apparent with age.

The typical features associated with PWS, such as intellectual disability and behavioural problems, emerge as the child develops. Approximately 90–100% of children with PWS will have delayed motor development.

After the NIPE

When a potential congenital abnormality is suspected it is essential that the MDT is involved in formulating a plan. Appropriate clinical decision-making is required to assess if the abnormality requires an urgent review by a neonatologist/ paediatrician or a referral to an appropriate specialist.

If a genetic problem is suspected, the infant should be examined by a clinical genetics specialist, who may be able to identify the underlying cause and initiate testing. Finding a genetic cause for the infant's problems will often have implications for other family members.

On transferring the infant to community care it is imperative to ensure that the parents are aware of their ongoing appointments and with whom. Relevant members of the MDT need to be informed and, if possible, telephone numbers and contacts for relevant support groups should be given to the parents.

A practitioner completing the NIPE should be confident in being able to recognise congenital abnormalities and take the appropriate action required for referral and follow-up. Liaison with other members of the MDT is essential when there is uncertainty. Any infant who presents with dysmorphic features and/or the potential presence of a congenital abnormality should be referred to a clinical geneticist. A geneticist will play a pivotal role in assisting the MDT to make a definitive diagnosis through detailed clinical assessment and ordering appropriate investigations. Accurate diagnosis not only is necessary for management of the infant, but will also be able to provide parents with further information about future risk.

With early detection of congenital anomalies, the NIPE practitioner can ensure that appropriate intervention, treatment and management can be initiated promptly.

Glossary

Amniocentesis: a small volume of amniotic fluid is removed under ultrasound guidance. Fetal cells are extracted and analysed.

Brachycephaly: characterised by a flattened area at the back of an infant's skull.

Chorionic villous sampling: a sample of placental tissue is obtained for genetic analysis.

Congenital: refers to existence at or before birth.

Consanguinity: when parents are related by blood.

Dysmorphic features: a difference in body structure. It can be an isolated finding in an otherwise normal individual, or it can be related to a congenital disorder.

Epicanthic folds: folds of skin across the inner corner of the eye.

Exomphalos: abdominal wall defect in which the abdominal organs remain outside the body, covered in a membrane.

Glossoptosis: a tongue that is situated further back than normal.

Hypotonia: decreased muscle tone leading to a floppy infant.

Karyotype: an individual's collection of chromosomes.

Macroglossia: abnormal enlargement of the tongue.

Microcephaly: the circumference of the head is smaller than usual.

Micrognathia: small lower jaw.

Palpebral fissures: the opening between the eyelids.

References

Abdilla, Y., Barbara, M.A. and Calleja-Agius, J. (2017). Prader–Willi syndrome: background and management. *Neonatal Network*, **36**(3): 134–41.

Bondy, C.A. (2007). Care of girls and women with Turner syndrome. *Journal of Clinical Endocrinology Metabolism*, **92**(1): 10–25.

Chitkara, E. (2016). Consanguineous marriages increase risk of congenital anomalies. *Biomedical Research*, **27**(1): 34–3.

David, R., Murdock, F.X., Donovan. S.C., Settera, C., Chandrasekharappa, N.B. and Bondy, C. (2017). Whole-exome sequencing for diagnosis of Turner syndrome: toward the next generation. *Journal of Clinical Endocrinology Metabolism*, **105**(5): 1529–37.

EUROCAT (2018). European Surveillance of Congenital Abnormalities. Available at: www.eurocat-network.eu/prenatalscreeninganddiagnosis/generalinformation/introduction (accessed 20 April 2018).

Lalani, S.R. (2017). Current genetic testing tools in neonatal medicine. *Paediatrics and Neonatology*, **58**: 111–21.

Loane, M., Morris, J.K., Addor, M., Arriola, L., Budd, J., Doray, B. et al. (2013). Twenty year trends in the prevalence of Down Syndrome and other trisomies in Europe: Impact of maternal age and prenatal screening. *European Journal of Human Genetics*, **27**: 27–33.

Oktay, K., Bedoschi, G., Berkowitz, K., Bronson, R., Kashani, B., McGovern, P. et al.

(2016). Fertility preservation in females with Turner syndrome: A comprehensive review and practical guidelines. *Journal of Pediatric and Adolescent Gynecology*, **29**: 409–16.

Office for National Statistics (2016). Birth by parents' characteristics in England and Wales: 2016. Available at: www.ons.gov.uk/peoplepopulationandcommunity/ birthsdeathsandmarriages/livebirths/bulletins/birthsbyparentscharacteristic sinenglandandwales/2016 (accessed 11 May 2018).

Public Health England (2018). *Newborn and Infant Examination Screening Standards*. Available at: www.gov.uk/government/publications/newborn-and-infant-physical-examination-programme-handbook/newborn-and-infant-physical-examination-screening-programme-handbook (accessed 26 April 2018).

Ranweiler, R. (2009). Assessment and care of the newborn with Down syndrome. *Advances in Neonatal Care*, **9** (1): 17–24.

Rennie, J.M. (2012). *Rennie and Robertson's Textbook of Neonatology*, 5th edn. Edinburgh: Churchill Livingstone.

Romano, A.A., Allanson, J.E., Dahlgren, J., Gelb, B.D., Hall, B., Pierpont, M. et al. (2010). Noonan syndrome: Clinical features, diagnosis, and management guidelines. *Paediatrics*, **126**: 746–59.

Royal College of Paediatrics and Child Health (2015). *Palate Examination: Identification of Cleft Palate in the Newborn-Best Practice Guide*. Available at www.rcpch. ac.uk/resources/palate-examination-identification-cleft-palate-newborn-best-practice-guide (accessed 10 May 2018).

Sadler, T.W. (2015). *Langman's Medical Embryology*, 13th edn. Philadelphia., PA: Wolters Kluwer.

Sinha, S., Miall, L. and Jardine, L. (2017). *Essential Neonatal Medicine*, 6th edn. London: Wiley Blackwell.

Vrijheid, M., Dolk, H., Stone, D., Abramsky, L., Alberman, E. and Scott, E.S. (2000). Socioeconomic inequalities in risk of congenital anomaly. *Archives of Disease in Childhood*, **82**: 349–52.

World Health Organization (2016). *Congenital anomalies. Factsheet*. Available at: www.who.int/mediacentre/factsheets/fs370/en (accessed 13 April 2018).

Zammit, M., Caruana, E. and Cassar, D. (2017). Beck–Weidemann syndrome review: A guide for neonatal nurses. *Neonatal Network*, **36**(3): 129–33.

Overview of the NIPE and appropriate and timely referral pathways

Anne Lomax and Claire Evans

Overview of the NIPE

The aim of the newborn and infant physical examination (NIPE) is to:

> identify and refer all babies born with congenital abnormalities of the heart, hips, eyes or testes, where these are detectable, within 72 hours of birth.

> further identify abnormalities that may be detected, at the second physical examination performed between 6 to 8 weeks of age.
>
> (Public Health England, 2018a, Section 1)

Timely and appropriate referral for a suspected anomaly found at the time of the examination is integral to the purpose of the diagnostic and treatment pathway, with the aim of improving overall outcome and the future wellbeing of the infant.

The aim of screening is to identify those in the population at greater risk of having a particular condition.

The aims of this chapter are to do the following:

- Outline the four screening elements of the NIPE screening programme standards and recommended timescales for specialist review
- Reaffirm the common conditions found on the newborn and infant physical examination covered in the previous chapters
- Provide a rationale as to the need for timely referral for the suspected anomaly
- Outline other findings at the examination where referral and treatment management are required.

First and foremost, any suitably trained practitioner undertaking the full newborn examination must be familiar with the local clinical guidelines and protocols, which will outline exclusion criteria for the examination. These should be available within the trust. This document is normally developed and published through collaboration between trust senior midwives and consultant neonatologists/paediatricians and written within the parameters of the trust's clinical governance standards. The document will normally be informed by the key 2018 Public Health England (2018a, 2018b) reference sources.

NIPE Programme Standards

See Public Health England (2018a).

NIPE Programme Handbook

See Public Health England (2018b).

NIPE Programme Service Specification No. 21

See Public Health England (2018a).

Examples of current trust guidelines for the NIPE can easily be found on the internet; however, the document usually has a standard structure.

Some guidelines will detail specific guidance on individual aspects of the examination and outline pathways of referral for each abnormality. A review date for the protocol will be set by the trust and will normally be updated between 3 and 5 years, or reviewed as new evidence or national guidance becomes available.

The NHS NIPE Screening Programme provides standards aligned to four of the most common conditions identified at the time of the newborn and infant examination. If undetected at birth or at the newborn and 6- to 8-week examination, the potential exists for long-term health sequelae and less favourable outcomes for the infant. Undetected congenital defects, such as critical heart defects, are life threatening and remain a significant cause of perinatal and infant mortality (Manzoni et al., 2017).

For an outline of the NIPE programme standards and recommended timely referrals see Public Health England (2018a).

The four screening elements of the NIPE screening programme are now revisited for confirmation of understanding.

Eyes

The ocular pathways are not completely developed at birth but mature progressively during the neonatal period. The central nervous system develops as the eye grows within the first weeks and months of birth. The myelin sheath that covers the nerve fibres of the ocular pathways does not mature until approximately 2 years of age. Moreover, focus or sharpness of vision in the eye develops rapidly in the early newborn period; this process reaches maturity around 3 years of age (Lomax, 2015).

It is for these reasons that it is crucial to establish the presence of the red reflex and recognise any ocular abnormalities early in the newborn, to prevent any interference with this development. In particular, unilateral cataract in the newborn presents a 'therapeutic window of opportunity' as little as 6 weeks after birth, and failure to treat this condition within this time frame can result in unilateral deprivation of the visual system. This impacts significantly on long-term rehabilitation of vision in the infant (Khokhar et al., 2018).

The examination should begin by reviewing the maternal health and obstetric records. A history of familial diseases, such as retinoblastoma, may necessitate a full examination of the fundus after birth (Orge and Grigorian, 2018). Other risk factors include: a family history of congenital cataracts, prematurity, maternal exposure to viruses in pregnancy such as rubella and syndromes such as trisomy 21 (Public Health England, 2018a). A suggested approach to the clinical examination of the eye can be found in Chapter 6A. The NHS NIPE Screening Programme Handbook (Public Health England, 2018b) also provides an appropriate evidence base for this approach.

Early intervention and prompt referral in cases where an abnormality has been detected are therefore crucial, and effective referral pathways must be in place to facilitate this. The revised national standards for the NHS NIPE Screening Programme (Public Heath England, 2018a) provide timescales that practitioners should follow to ensure timely interventions and early commencement of an effective treatment pathway for babies who have a positive screen for eye abnormalities.

Heart

At birth most term babies will experience an uneventful transition from fetal to postnatal life. The main circulatory and pulmonary changes occur within the first few moments; however, it can take up to 6 weeks after birth for true physiological transition to be complete (Askin, 2009).

Around 1 in 200 babies may have a heart problem and these problems are divided into critical and non-critical categories (Public Health England, 2018b). Many cardiac defects are not discernible in the early neonatal period, so practitioners must be competent in continuous assessment of the infant throughout this period and be able to recognise early symptoms of serious cardiac disease. They must understand the importance of prompt referral in order to implement the most appropriate treatment, and to minimise neonatal mortality and morbidity that can arise from such defects (Bedford and Lomax, 2015). Understanding the theory behind the development of the heart and lungs is essential if the practitioner is to be effective in early recognition of cardiac problems. Moreover, a thorough review of the maternal history and family history is essential in anticipating cardiac disease in the infant (see Chapter 6b). Risk factors for congenital cardiac disease can be found in the NHS NIPE Programme Handbook (Public Health England, 2018b).

Today many babies leave hospital within a few hours of birth and consequently there are limitations to performing an early newborn examination. Cardiac murmurs are considered to be the hallmark of cardiac disease; however, the early examination of the infant may not reveal a murmur at this stage. Some babies may demonstrate subtle signs of illness only in the neonatal period and parents who communicate that their infant is not feeding well or is 'not quite right' must be taken seriously because this may be an indication of early warning signs of congenital cardiac disease. The infant must be examined closely with this in mind (Bedford and Lomax, 2015).

In a significant number of cases, more obvious symptoms do not develop until after discharge from hospital (Almawasini et al., 2017). For example, a murmur arising from a ventricular septal defect may not be apparent at birth, but develop over the first few weeks of life. The NIPE practitioner should ensure that, on discharge, the parents have information detailing what to do if the infant becomes unwell, and also that they have easy access to healthcare professionals. The importance of attendance at the 6- to 8-week check must be emphasised (Lomax, 2015). The competent practitioner must therefore be alert to the features in both the history and the examination that may indicate a congenital heart defect.

In some cases, a murmur can be present in an otherwise healthy infant at birth with no associated clinical symptoms. Usually this is due to the considerable circulatory changes that occur after birth, and the benign murmur that is produced turns out to be transient in nature (Gladman, 2012). Abnormal heart sounds, however, even in the asymptomatic infant, must be referred to a senior paediatrician urgently (see Chapter 6B).

Pulse oximetry has been shown to improve early detection of congenital heart disease in newborn babies by identifying those with low saturations before symptoms have manifested themselves (Almawasini et al., 2018). Other serious conditions that manifest in the same way can also be detected, such as sepsis or pneumonia (Manzoni et al., 2017). The UK National Screening Committee (NSC) have not yet published standards on the cardiac examination or included the routine use of pulse oximetry as part of the NIPE examination. In 2015 they supported a pilot study looking at the feasibility of rolling out newborn pulse oximetry screening and the possible impact of implementing this practice on the NHS. The UK NSC has yet to make a decision with regard to any national roll-out of newborn pulse oximetry screening.

Hips

Developmental dysplasia of the hip (DDH) is a term that covers a range of developmental abnormalities of the femoral head and acetabulum. The abnormal hip joint, if undetected, can cause degenerative joint disease and permanent disability in later life.

In the UK the national NIPE Programme (Public Health England, 2018a, Section 6.2) outlines certain risk factors that may alert the examiner to the presence of an abnormal hip(s) in the newborn. They also state that the newborn hips should be examined clinically through observation and by performing Ortolani and Barlow's stability manoeuvres, within 72 hours of birth (Public Health England, 2018a).

Although there is some controversy around the reliability of this the justification for including Ortolani and Barlow's manoeuvres in the current UK screening policy remains, and some studies have shown that, in experienced hands, these manoeuvres performed soon after birth are capable of identifying some cases of unstable or dislocated hips earlier than they would have otherwise been identified (Sulaiman et al., 2011). Universal ultrasound screening of suspected DDH is still seen as the gold standard; however, it is not regarded as cost-effective to perform on all babies and so only those with a positive test, or a negative test and positive risk factors, will undergo screening in the UK (Public Health England, 2018a).

Early identification and prompt referral for DDH are essential, if DDH remains undetected, then the inevitable joint pathology that follows will significantly impair walking and possibly require surgical intervention. Early non-surgical intervention, with abduction of the hip in a Pavlik harness or similar abduction brace, will promote correct alignment and stabilisation of the hip joint (Shipman et al., 2006).

The NHS NIPE Screening Programme Handbook (Public Health England, 2018b) also provides an appropriate evidence base for hip examination. The revised national standards for the NHS NIPE Screening Programme (Public Health England, 2018a) provide a referral process that practitioners can follow to ensure timely interventions and early commencement of effective treatment.

Parents can access support, information leaflets and visual resources from the STEPS charity – a national charity for lower limb conditions available at: www.steps-charity.org.uk/conditions/talipes-clubfoot.

Testes

Chromosomes and gonads are both key to the determination of the gender of a neonate. In the normal development of a male fetus, the testes develop in the abdominal cavity. At approximately 28 weeks' gestation, they will descend through the internal inguinal ring into the inguinal canal, and then to the external inguinal ring and finally into the scrotum.

It is normal for this process in a full-term infant to be completed by birth; however, in the preterm infant it is likely that the testes may not be present in the scrotum (Gordon, 2015).

Cryptorchidism is a term describing a condition in which one or both testes fail to descend from the abdominal cavity; it occurs in between 2% and 6% of males at term; however 70% of these will descend normally by 12 months of age (Acerini et al., 2009).

There are certain risk factors to be aware of when reviewing the antenatal, intrapartum and immediate postnatal history of an infant with suspected cryptorchidism:

- A first-degree family history of cryptorchidism (infant's father or sibling)
- Low birth weight
- Small for gestational age or preterm birth

(Public Health England, 2018b, section 7.2)

At examination a range of findings may be present. A single palpable undescended testicle or a single impalpable undescended testicle requires referral to a paediatrician or in line with local trust polices. Bilateral palpable or impalpable undescended testes require urgent if not emergency referral or as directed by local trust policy.

Although it is rare to find bilateral undescended testes, such findings must be acted on promptly because this condition carries a significant increased risk of testicular cancer, infertility, hypospadias and testicular torsion (Public Health England, 2018b). In addition this may be associated with ambiguous genitalia or underlying metabolic disease such as congenital adrenal hyperplasia (CAH) or androgen insensitivity syndrome (AIS).

CAH is characterised by a recessive inherited enzyme deficiency, which causes a life-threatening adrenal or salt-wasting crisis through impaired production of aldosterone. In addition overstimulation of the sex hormone testosterone causes virilised female genitalia and can result in difficulties with gender assignment on examination. Emergency referral is required to prevent dehydration, which can occur quickly (Knowles et al., 2011).

AIS is a disorder that arises from the complete or partial resistance to the biological actions of androgens in an XY male. This results in the body developing phenotypically as a female. The accompanying ambiguous genitalia again make it difficult for gender assignment at birth (Hughes et al., 2012).

In these cases establishment of a diagnosis and reaching a decision on gender assignment are key elements of the examination. Once again, early intervention and prompt referral, when an abnormality has been detected, is crucial and effective referral pathways must be in place to facilitate this. The revised national standards for the NIPE Screening Programme (Public Health England, 2018a) provide a process practitioners can follow to ensure timely interventions and early commencement of an effective treatment pathway for babies who have a positive screen for abnormality of the testes.

Other clinical findings/pathology that require referral

The NIPE Screening Programme Standards (Public Health England, 2018a) recommend the referral of newborns with screen-positive findings on the four screening elements of the NIPE examination, but in line with local policies the timely and appropriate referral of any other abnormality found during the rest of the NIPE may also be required. There are a number of other significant findings that require the NIPE practitioner to have the infant reviewed and arrange referral to the appropriate specialism. There are many normal variants found in the newborn that may be genetic in origin. Mothers often examine their newborn and may have already identified a familial variant, e.g. a cutaneous lesion that a sibling had at birth.

This section addresses some of those findings that are significant and even life threatening which require review, investigation and treatment. If an abnormality is suspected by the NIPE practitioner, the newborn must be reviewed by a senior member of the paediatric medical team to confirm or negate the findings. If confirmed, then a referral management plan can be put in place to ensure referral in a timely manner to the appropriate specialist team. A framework for the conditions listed with referral specialism, timescales and additional educational resources for healthcare professionals and parents are provided in Table 8.1.

Antenatal hydronephrosis

Antenatal hydronephrosis is defined as dilatation of the renal pelvis collecting system. It is bilateral in 20–40% of cases (Chen et al., 2010). This anomaly is usually detected on the fetal anomaly scan. The condition can be unilateral or bilateral. From diagnosis, the pregnancy is usually managed jointly by a fetal medicine consultant and the paediatric urology or nephrology specialist. All pregnancies diagnosed with hydronephrosis will require antenatal and postnatal ultrasound surveillance. Parents are provided with the opportunity to discuss the postnatal management plan and ongoing monitoring of the condition, as well as possible treatment options if they become necessary. Newborns with antenatally diagnosed complex renal pathology will be managed from birth by the neonatal unit.

The newborn with hydronephrosis is followed up with a repeat ultrasound scan in the postnatal period. The NIPE practitioner should ensure that the renal ultrasound appointment is made before discharge and a postnatal appointment also made with the paediatric urology or nephrology team. The first postnatal renal ultrasound is usually performed at age 1 week with a repeat scan at age 6 weeks depending on local hydronephrosis guidelines. Further postnatal investigation may be required, e.g. micturating cystourethrogram (Langstaff and Mallik, 2014). Hydronephrosis is graded by the anteroposterior diameter measurement on serial antenatal scans, ranging from less than 9 mm indicating mild dilatation in the third trimester to severe with an anteroposterior diameter of more than 15 mm (Psooy and Pike, 2008).

The severity of the antenatal hydronephrosis can in some cases indicate further renal pathology, e.g. posterior urethral valves, vesicoureteric junction obstruction or vesicoureteric reflux (VUS) (Hothi et al., 2009; Chen et al., 2010;

Table 8.1 Referral specialisms and timescales

Abnormality	Referral specialisms	Timescale for referral	Additional resources
Congenital cataracts Abnormality of the eyes	Senior paediatric medical team Consultant ophthalmologist/ paediatric ophthalmology service	Attendance at an assessment appointment by 2 weeks of age (Public Health England, 2018b)	www.gov.uk/government/ publications/newborn-and-infant-physical-examination-screening-standards www.gov.uk/government/ publications/newborn-and-infant-physical-examination-programme-handbook www.gov.uk/government/ publications/newborn-and-infant-physical-examination-screening-standards www.e-lfh.org.uk/?s=examination+of +the+newborn
Congenital cardiac defect	Senior paediatric medical team Paediatrician with expertise in cardiology Regional paediatric cardiac unit	Senior paediatrician review (urgency depends on suspected condition), but review is recommended before discharge home (Public Health England, 2018b)	www.gov.uk/government/ publications/newborn-and-infant-physical-examination-screening-standards www.gov.uk/government/ publications/newborn-and-infant-physical-examination-programme-handbook www.gov.uk/government/ publications/newborn-and-infant-physical-examination-screening-standards www.e-lfh.org.uk/?s=examination+of +the+newborn

Table 8.1 Continued

Abnormality	Referral specialisms	Timescale for referral	Additional resources
Developmental dysplasia of the hip	Senior paediatric medical team Consultant orthopaedic surgeon	Attendance for a specialist hip ultrasound within 2 weeks of age (Public Health England, 2018b) Babies with a negative screening test on NIPE but with identified risk factors should have an assessment by specialist hip ultrasound before 6 weeks of age (Public Health England, 2018b)	www.gov.uk/government/ publications/newborn-and-infant-physical-examination-screening-standards www.gov.uk/government/ publications/newborn-and-infant-physical-examination-programme-handbook www.gov.uk/government/ publications/newborn-and-infant-physical-examination-screening-standards www.e-lfh.org.uk/?s=examination+of +the+newborn www.e-lfh.org.uk/programmes/nhs-screening-programmes
Bilateral undescended testes	Senior paediatric medical team Paediatrician with expertise in urology/paediatric urology team	Babies with bilateral undescended testes detected on NIPE should be seen within 24 hours of the examination	www.gov.uk/government/ publications/newborn-and-infant-physical-examination-screening-standards www.gov.uk/government/ publications/newborn-and-infant-physical-examination-programme-handbook www.gov.uk/government/ publications/newborn-and-infant-physical-examination-screening-standards www.e-lfh.org.uk/?s=examination+of +the+newborn

| Sick newborn | Senior paediatric medical team | **Urgent** (if infant at high risk and on a NEWS chart, score indicates review time by senior paediatric medical team (15–30 min) | www.bapm.org/news/launch-atain-elearning-programme
www.e-lfh.org.uk/programmes/avoiding-term-admissions-into-neonatal-units/
www.nice.org.uk/guidance/cg149/resources/neonatal-infection-early-onset-antibiotics-for-prevention-and-treatment-pdf-35109579233221
https://pathways.nice.org.uk/pathways/early-onset-neonatal-infection
www.mumandinfantacademy.co.uk/learn/could-this-be-neonatal-sepsis
www.mumandbabyacademy.co.uk/learn/group-b-strep_mf |
| Cleft palate | Senior paediatric medical team
Local service cleft lip and palate specialist nurse | **Urgent** review by senior paediatrician before discharge
Urgent referral to local cleft lip and palate specialist nurse and reviewed before discharge | www.clapa.com
www.rcpch.ac.uk/system/files/protected/page/Cleft%20palate%20best%20practice%20guide%20FINAL_1.pdf |

Table 8.1 Continued

Abnormality	Referral specialisms	Timescale for referral	Additional resources
Tongue-tie	Senior paediatric medical team Lactation consultant/infant feeding coordinator	Referral to lactation consultant/infant feeding coordinator before discharge For severe tongue-tie refer to paediatric medical team and lactation consultant/infant feeding coordinator before discharge Referral to frenulotomy clinic or ear, nose and throat (ENT) department (if indicated) within 2 weeks of age	www.tongue-tie.org.uk/tongue-tie-information.html www.nhs.uk/conditions/tongue-tie www.unicef.org.uk/babyfriendly/baby-friendly-resources/support-for-parents/tongue-tie www.nice.org.uk/guidance/ipg149/resources/division-of-ankyloglossia-tongue-tie-for-breastfeeding-pdf-304342237 www.mumandbabyacademy.co.uk/learn/tongue-tie-and-breastfeeding www.ilearn.rcm.org.uk/course/view.php?id=165 (password access required)
Antenatal hydronephrosis	Paediatric urology or nephrology team Ultrasound department	Referral to paediatric urology/nephrology service Follow-up renal ultrasound scan appointment at 1 week and 6 weeks of age	
Polydactyly and/or syndactyly	Senior paediatric medical team Paediatric plastic surgery team	Referral to paediatric plastic surgery team	https://benthamopen.com/FULLTEXT/TOORTHJ-6-14 https://journals.lww.com/prsgo/fulltext/2017/11000/Genetic_Overview_of_Syndactyly_and_Polydactyly.8.aspx www.orthobullets.com/hand/6079/polydactyly-of-hand

Congenital talipes	Senior paediatric medical team Paediatric orthopaedic team Paediatric physiotherapy team	**Urgent** referral to the paediatric orthopaedic team and reviewed before discharge	www.steps-charity.org.uk/conditions/talipes-clubfoot www.orthobullets.com/pediatrics/4062/clubfoot-congenital-talipes-equinovarus
Dysmorphism	Senior paediatric medical team		www.downs-syndrome.org.uk www.soft.org.uk

Langstaff and Mallik, 2014). Controversy exists surrounding the use of post-natal prophylactic antibiotics for the newborn (Psooy and Pike, 2008; Langstaff and Mallik, 2014), but they may be prescribed on an individual basis depending on the degree of dilatation until all investigations have been completed to reduce the risk of a urinary tract infection (UTI) that may cause renal scarring.

Observation of urinary output in the postnatal period will give some indication of renal function. However, a normal stream does not completely exclude the presence of posterior urethral valves. Parents of newborns with prenatal hydronephrosis should be advised before discharge about possible symptoms in their infant that may be indicative of a urinary tract infection and to see their GP urgently. See Table 8.2 for possible symptoms of a neonatal UTI. The condition will be managed jointly by the paediatric urology team and the GP in the postnatal period.

Cleft palate

A cleft lip and palate anomaly is usually detected on the fetal anomaly scan but not always. Recent data from the Cleft Lip and Palate Association (CLAPA) suggest that 91% of cleft lip and palate are detected at the fetal anomaly scan (see www.clapa.com). However, the isolated cleft palate is not detected prenatally. A submucous cleft is particularly difficult to identify. The rate of missed isolated cleft palates at the time of the newborn examination was disturbing high prompting the Royal College of Paediatrics and Child Health (RCPCH) to produce national guidance (RCPCH, 2014) on how to correctly examine the palate using a light source and tongue depressor, usually in the form of a sterile, single use-only wooden spatula. Digital palpation alone of the oral cavity is not effective in detecting a cleft palate. Close inspection and full visualisation of both the hard and soft palate are essential to exclude a cleft.

A feeding history of persistent vomiting down the nose can be a symptom of a cleft palate and is a question that should be asked as part of the feeding behaviour of the newborn. Oral challenges will present in the newborn with a

Table 8.2 Possible symptoms of a neonatal urinary tract infection
Poor feeding
Vomiting
Diarrhoea
Unstable temperature – hyper- and hypothermia
Listlessness
Offensive smelling urine

cleft palate. An urgent referral to the local cleft lip and palate specialist nurse is essential to ensure that feeding challenges are resolved and parents feel reassured and confident in feeding their infant before discharge. The cleft lip and palate special nurse, alongside the lactation consultant/infant feeding coordinator, will advise mothers on correct positioning to help establish and maintain breastfeeding. Provision and advice on special feeding bottles and teats for formula feeding and expressed breast milk are also offered by this specialist service. Surgical repair of the cleft palate is usually performed while the infant is aged 6–12 months. A support network from the team and charity CLAPA can provide parents with useful information at www.clapa.com. Visual educational resources can also be found on this website.

Any delay in the diagnosis and referral into treatment to the local cleft lip and palate team can impact on the health and development of the newborn. In the first instance, feeding difficulties from an undiagnosed cleft palate will result in weight loss and associated problems, e.g. jaundice. In the long term an undiagnosed cleft, including the submucous cleft, can affect speech development and hearing. It is essential that the mouth and palate are afforded the same degree of inspection at the 6- to 8-week infant examination.

Tongue-tie

Tongue-tie or ankyloglossia is a congenital anomaly in which the frenulum positioned on the underside of the tongue is short and limits the mobility and function of the tongue (National Institute for Health and Care Excellence [NICE], 2005). The incidence is reported as 3–7% of births (Finigan, 2014). The short frenulum is usually found on examination of the mouth during the NIPE. There may be a history of feeding problems with poor attachment when breastfeeding. It is important that the NIPE practitioner takes a full feeding history to establish the true impact of the condition on feeding. Referral to the trust lactation consultant or infant feeding coordinator may be required to fully assess the degree of tongue-tie. Referral to the local frenulotomy service may be required for surgical division of the frenulum, in clinically significant cases, to improve mobility of the tongue. The degree of tongue-tie can vary from mild to severe. Mild tongue-tie involves the tongue being restricted by a thin mucous membrane whereas severe is when the tongue is completely fused to the mouth floor (NICE, 2005). The NICE (2005) produced guidance in support of the division of tongue-tie for breastfeeding.

Feeding challenges can present for the newborn with moderate-to-severe tongue-tie, which includes restricted tongue function, excessive wind resulting from an irregular sucking pattern, reflux, weight loss and general fractiousness when feeding (Association of Tongue-tie Practitioners [ATP], see www.nhs.uk/conditions/tongue-tie). Mothers may experience nipple pain, poor lactation and an overall dissatisfaction with breastfeeding, resulting in exhaustion and opting to feed the newborn formula milk. However, if sufficiently problematic, this condition may also present feeding challenges for the formula-fed newborn.

Tongue-tie can be a great source of concern and stress to parents when feeding challenges present. Healthcare professionals involved in newborn care must provide the essential information and support that parents require during the perinatal period after diagnosis of this anomaly. Prompt referral for an assessment and breastfeeding support from a lactation specialist are vital to ensure that breastfeeding is not disrupted and an onward referral for frenulotomy is indeed justified. The ATP provides a video resource to assess feeding ability with tongue-tie (see www.tongue-tie.org.uk/tongue-tie-information.html).

The UNICEF United Kingdom Baby Friendly Initiative provides information and support for parents of babies with tongue-tie.

The website also provides results from recent studies conducted internationally which can help inform advice and support provided by healthcare practitioners to parents.

Foot abnormalities

There are various forms of congenital foot abnormalities that involve defined parts of the foot (Paton and Davies, 2015). These can be positional or structural in nature, and the treatment and outcome varies greatly depending on this. In rare cases the foot abnormality may be in addition to other anomalies forming a more complex condition. Parents can also access support, information leaflets and visual resources from the STEPS charity (www.steps-charity.org.uk/conditions/talipes-clubfoot). It is outwith the remit of this chapter to explore the complete spectrum of congenital abnormalities, but see Chapter 6E. There is some debate about whether there is an association between clubfoot and DDH; however, it is not a national risk factor for the screening of DDH under the national NIPE Programme Standards for DDH (Public Health England, 2018a). There is, however, more evidence to support the association between DDH and calcaneovalgus foot postures, although this is also not a national risk factor – the NIPE practitioner should, however, refer to their local guidelines.

Polydactyly and syndactyly

Examination of the hands and feet is conducted as part of the NIPE to exclude the presence of supplementary digits, and fusion of or abnormal positioning of digits. This can be unilateral or bilateral, present as syndromic or non-syndromic.

Polydactyly and syndactyly can be a source of concern and stress to parents and the family. Referral to the paediatric plastic surgery team is often necessary for functional as well as aesthetic reasons. It is important that the NIPE practitioner and the paediatric medical team fully explain the extent of the abnormality, and that the referral to the paediatric plastic surgery team is made in a timely manner, to ensure entry of the infant into a treatment pathway that will maximise the functionality of the limb(s) in the long term.

Sacral dimple

The presence of an isolated sacral dimple in the newborn is a common finding during the NIPE. In most cases the dimple does not represent any clinical pathology and is essentially benign. In very rare cases the dimple may indicate an underlying spinal cord or spine anomaly such as spina bifida occulta.

The dimple can be defined as simple or complex (Wilson et al., 2016). The lesion is diameter and position dependent, and its appearance will determine the need for ultrasonography to assess the depth of the anomaly and the spinal cord. The simple sacral dimple should be shallow and the base easily seen and defined as a single midline dimple less than 5 mm in diameter and less than 25 mm from the anus (Wilson et al., 2016). It should not present with any skin lesions, such as a hair tuft or haemangioma close to the dimple area (Lewis, 2014).

The complex sacral dimple is deep and associated with other clinical findings. Review by a senior paediatrician is required if it cannot be established that the dimple is blind ended. If ultrasonography is required it is usually performed before age 3 months (Lewis, 2016). Magnetic resonance imaging (MRI) may be indicated as another form of diagnostic investigation. Controversy surrounds the use of ultrasonography and its use for diagnostic purposes in the absence of any neurological involvement (Chern et al., 2012). Lee et al. (2007) reported an incidence of sacral dimple in 0.5% ($n = 26$) from 5440 live births. Only six infants had a hair tuft and four had ultrasonography or an MRI with no abnormality detected; of the 16 infants followed up none had any neurological impairment.

The sick newborn

Most newborns will have a normal NIPE screen. However, the examination does not afford any margin for complacency. The NIPE practitioner must be constantly on the alert to identify the sick newborn. This subject is addressed in more detail in Chapter 6. In relation to appropriate and timely referral, it is vital that any infant giving cause for concern at the NIPE must be reviewed urgently by a senior paediatrician. Early onset neonatal infection remains a significant cause of mortality and morbidity in the newborn population (NICE, 2012). History taking and dialogue with the midwifery staff are implicit to the NIPE (Evans, 2015) and may identify the newborn at risk of early onset sepsis.

The newborn early warning system (NEWS) observation chart is used for any newborn with risk factors that warrant increased surveillance in the immediate newborn period (Roland et al., 2010, British Association of Perinatal Medicine

[BAPM], 2015). BAPM (2015) have developed a newborn early warning trigger and track (NEWTT) practice framework.

If an infant with risk factors and on the NEWS chart, the NIPE practitioner must review the documented observations. In addition they must ensure that the observation period on the chart is complete and that observations are within normal parameters before a discharge home recommendation is made. If there is any cause for concern and no NEWS chart in place at the time of the NIPE, then it is good practice to start one. The score given will indicate the escalation need and response time to review required from the paediatric medical team.

Clinical signs of early onset infection in the newborn can be subtle. It is therefore vital that the NIPE practitioner can recognise the newborn that is potentially infected. The newborn must be treated as such until diagnostic investigations confirm or negate any infection. It is helpful for the NIPE practitioner to be aware of the NICE (2012) guideline on early onset neonatal sepsis which signposts the red flag symptoms of sepsis in the newborn.

THINK POINT

You are about to perform the NIPE on an infant who is 39 weeks' gestation and 26 hours of age. The midwife comments that the infant has been sleepy and disinterested in breastfeeding overnight. The infant is not on a NEWS chart and there are no risk factors for early onset infection. The mother comments that the infant is much sleepier than her last infant.

You notice the infant to be pale and tachypnoeic with nasal flaring. You perform a set of observations:

> Respiratory rate 88 beats/min
> Temperature 36.2°C
> Oxygen saturations 84%
> Heart rate 154 beats/min
> Capillary refill 3 seconds with fair perfusion

What will your immediate actions be?
What information will you provide to the mother?

Pulse oximetry may be one of the physiological parameter measurements on the NEWS chart. It is an extremely useful and quick tool to establish the infant's oxygen saturation reading and heart rate. A recent study by Mikrou et al. (2017) reported that 40% of trusts in England are performing pulse oximetry screening before discharge to aid the detection of critical congenital heart defects (CCHDs). An abnormal pulse oximetry result may be the first indication that the infant is unwell. Equally most trusts perform 'target' pulse oximetry on the sick newborn found to be unwell at the time of the NIPE or any other time on the postnatal ward. As previously discussed CCHDs can be asymptomatic, but in most cases hypoxaemia is present and detectable by pulse oximetry. Low oxygen saturation levels demand urgent review by a senior paediatrician and immediate transfer to the neonatal unit.

Parental communication and support

Parents must be given information before the examination and for screening: the *Screening Tests for You and Your Baby* booklet (Public Health England, 2018c) should be provided. The outcome of the NIPE and accurate appropriate information should be discussed about any abnormality is detected. Anomalies that require specialist clinic appointments should be made before the discharge of the newborn where possible. Anomaly-specific local trust information leaflets can be helpful for parents and should be given where these are available. It is also important for parents to know the timeline from discharge to clinic appointment. In some cases this can help reiterate the importance of the condition and the need to attend the appointment with their infant.

It is also important to advise parents that some problems may not be evident at the time of the NIPE. As discussed earlier advice must be given to parents at the time of the NIPE on possible signs of illness and points of contact. Parents must also be informed at the time of the NIPE that a further 6- to 8-week examination will be performed by the GP or other suitability trained practitioner. The health visitor will arrange for the appointment.

Parents should also be advised that, when an antenatal anomaly diagnosis is made, the antenatal scan results will be shared and reported to the National Congenital Anomaly and Rare Disease Registration (NCARDRS; Public Health England, 2017). NCARDRS collate data nationally on all fetal anomalies and those diagnosed postnatally.

Governance issues

It is vital to the referral pathway process that diagnostic and treatment appointments are tracked and monitored through the referral pathway and attendance at appointments recorded. This gives reassurance of the screening or clinical pathway. Parents who do not bring their infant to an appointment must be offered another appointment in line with the local trust non-attendance – 'did not attend' (DNA) or 'was not brought' (WNB) policy. The usual local policy is that after three DNAs a patient is referred back to the GP. However, in the instance of newborns and children, persistent DNA to appointments merits consideration as a safeguarding issue, and must be acted on in line with local safeguarding referral procedures.

The NIPE SMART IT system should be used to record and track appointments for all four screening elements, in line with local arrangements; other referral appointments under the 'rest of physical examination' should also be recorded. Outcomes from referrals for the four screening elements can be entered on the NIPE SMART system by way of the management plan arising from the referral appointment. The system provides local data and audit trail. The system can then be monitored locally to ensure the DNA-to-appointment rate is kept to a minimum and all followed up. Every trust using NIPE SMART should have a NIPE lead in post to monitor both NIPE SMART failsafe and the overall NIPE service (NHS Service Specification No. 21 2017/18). All local newborn referral pathways should be regularly reviewed to ensure the processes are evidence based and include contemporary national guidance or policy. Local failsafe processes should be in place to ensure that the referral processes are robust. It is essential that the NIPE practitioner is familiar with the trust's policies, guidelines or standard operating procedures in relation to the NIPE.

Referral to specialist follow-up appointments should be made where possible before discharge of the infant. The timely appointment will ensure that the infant enters the referral pathway as soon as possible, in line with the NHS NIPE Programme standards timescales (Public Health England, 2018a) where a referral is necessary. Significant delay may result in short- and long-term sequelae, or can be life threatening, particularly with undetected serious cardiac defects.

Adherence to guidelines and timescales must be observed to ensure appropriate and timely referral for further diagnostic investigations or treatment pathways, to maximise a successful outcome for the newborn.

References

Acerini, C.L., Miles, H.L., Dunger, D.B. et al. (2009). The descriptive epidemiology of congenital and acquired cryptorchidism in a UK infant cohort. *Archives of Diseases in Childhood*, **94**, 868–72.

Almawasini, A.M., Hanafi, H.K., Madkhali, H.K. and Majrashi, N.B. (2017). Effectiveness of the critical congenital heart disease screening program for early diagnosis of cardiac abnormalities in newborn infants. *Saudi Medical Journal*, **38**: 1019–24.

Askin, D. (2009). Fetal-to-neonatal transition: what is normal and what is not? Part 1. The physiology of transition. *Neonatal Network*, **28**(3): 33–6.

Bedford, C.D. and Lomax, A. (2015). Cardiovascular and respiratory assessment of the infant. In: *Examination of the Newborn: An Evidence Based Guide*, 2nd edn. London: Wiley, pp. 32–70.

British Association of Perinatal Medicine (2015). Newborn Early Warning Trigger and Track (NEWTT). A Framework for Practice. Available at: www.bapm.org/sites/default/files/files/NEWTT%20framework%20final.pdf (accessed March 2018).

Chen, Y., Lin, V.C. and Yu, T.J. (2010). Antenatal hydronephrosis. *Urology Science*, **21**: 109–12.

Chern, J.J., Kirkman, J.L., Shannon, C.N., Tubbs, R.S., Stone, J.D., Royal, S.A. et al. (2012). Use of lumbar ultrasonography to detect occult spinal dysraphism. *Journal Neurosurgery in Pediatrics*, **9**: 274–9.

Evans, C. (2015). History taking and the newborn examination: an evolving perspective. In: *Examination of the Newborn: An Evidence Based Guide*, 2nd edn. London: Wiley, pp. 1–31.

Finigan, V. (2014). Tongue tied. *Midwives*, **3**: 48–9.

Gladman, G. (2012). Management of asymptomatic heart murmurs. *Paediatrics and Child Health*, **23**(2): 64–8.

Gordon, M. (2015). Examination of the newborn abdomen and genitalia. In: *Examination of the Newborn: An Evidence Based Guide*, 2nd edn. London: Wiley, pp. 124–41.

Hothi, D.K., Wade, A.S., Gilbert, R. and Winyard, P.J.D. (2009). Mild fetal renal pelvis dilatation – much ado about nothing? *Clinical Journal American Society of Nephrology*, **4**: 168–77.

Hughes, I.A., Davies, J.D., Bunch, T.I., Paterski, V., Mastroyannopoulou, K. and MacDougall, J. (2012). Androgen insensitivity syndrome. *The Lancet*, **380**; 1419–28.

Khokhar, S., Jose, C. P., Sihota, R. and Midah, N. (2018). Unilateral congenital cataract: Clinical profile and presentation. *Journal of Clinical Ophthalmology and Strabismus*, **55**: 107–12.

Knowles, R.L., Oerton, J.M., Kahlid, J.M., Hindmarsh, P. and Kelnar, C. (2011). Clinical outcome of congenital adrenal hyperplasia (CAH) one year following diagnosis: A UK wide study. *Archives of Disease in Childhood*, **96**(Suppl 1): A27.

Langstaff, C. and Mallik, M. (2014). Antenatally detected urinary tract abnormalities (AUTA). *Paediatrics and Child Health*, **24**: 7.

Lee, A.C.W., Kwong, N.S. and Wong, Y.C. (2007). Management of sacral dimples detected on routine newborn examination: A case series and review. *Hong Kong Journal of Paediatrics*, **12**: 93–5.

Lewis, M.L. (2014). A comprehensive newborn examination: Part II. Skin, trunk, extremities, neurologic. *American Family Physician*, **90**: 5.

Lomax, A. (2015). *Examination of the Newborn: An Evidence-based Guide*, 2nd edn. Chichester: Wiley Blackwell.

Manzoni, P., Martin, G.R., Luna, M.S., Mestrovic, J., Simeoni, U., Zimmermann, L. and Ewer, A.K. (2017). Pulse oximetry screening for critical congenital heart defects: A European consensus statement. *The Lancet and Adolescent Health*, **1**(2): 88–90.

Mickrou, P., Singh, A. and Ewer, A.K. (2017). Pulse oximetry screening for critical congenital heart defects: A repeat UK national survey. *Archives of Diseases in Childhood, Fetal Neonatal Edition*, **0**: 1.

National Institute for Health and Care Excellence (NICE) (2005). *Division of Ankyloglossia (Tongue-tie) for Breastfeeding*. London: NICE. Available at: www.nice.org.uk/guidance/ipg149/resources/division-of-ankyloglossia-tongue-tie-for-breastfeeding-pdf-304342237 (accessed March 2018).

National Institute for Health and Care Excellence (2012). Antibiotics for early-onset neonatal infection. Antibiotics for the prevention and treatment of early-onset neonatal infection (CG 149) London: NICE Available at: www.nice.org.uk/guidance/cg149/resources/neonatal-infection-early-onset-antibiotics-for-prevention-and-treatment-pdf-35109579233221 (accessed April 2018).

Orge, F.H. and Grigorian, F. (2018). Examination and Common Problems of the Neonatal Eye. Obgynkey Available at: https://obgynkey.com/examination-and-common-problems-of-the-neonatal-eye (accessed May 2018).

Paton, R. and Davies, N. (2015). Developmental dysplasia of the hip and abnormalities of the foot. In: *Examination of the Newborn: An Evidence Based Guide*, 2nd edn. London: Wiley pp. 142–70.

Psooy, K. and Pike, J. (2008). Investigation and management of antenatally detected hydronephrosis. *Canadian Urological Association Journal*. Approved CUA Guidelines.

Public Health England (2017). National *Congenital Anomaly and Rare Disease Registration Service (NCARDRS) Guidance*. Available at: www.gov.uk/guidance/the-national-congenital-anomaly-and-rare-disease-registration-service-ncardrs (accessed April 2018).

Public Health England (2018a). *NHS Newborn Physical and Infant Examination Programme. NIPE Programme Standards*. Available at: www.gov.uk/government/publications/newborn-and-infant-physical-examination-screening-standards (accessed May 2018).

Public Health England (2018b). *NHS Newborn Physical and Infant Examination Programme. NIPE Programme Handbook*. Available at: www.gov.uk/government/publications/newborn-and-infant-physical-examination-programme-handbook/newborn-and-infant-physical-examination-screening-programme-handbook (accessed May 2018).

Public Health England (2018c). *NHS Fetal Anomaly Screening Programme (FASP) Fetal Anomaly Programme Standards*. Available at: www.gov.uk/government/publications/fetal-anomaly-screening-programme-standards/fetal-anomaly-screening-standards-valid-for-data-collected-from-1-april-2018 (accessed May 2018).

Roland, D., Madar, J. and Connolly, G. (2010). The Newborn Early Warning (NEW) System: Development of an at-risk infant intervention system. *Infant*, **6**(4): 116–19.

Royal College of Paediatricians and Child Health (2014). *Palate Examination: Identification of cleft palate in the newborn*. London: RCPCH. Available at: www.rcpch.ac.uk/system/files/protected/page/Cleft%20palate%20best%20practice%20guide%20FINAL_1.pdf (accessed March 2018).

Shipman, S.A., Halfand, M., Moyer, V.A. and Yawn, B.P. (2006). Screening for developmental dysplasia of the Hip: A systematic literature review for the US Preventive Services Task Force. *Pediatrics*, **117**(3): e557–76.

Sulaiman, A.R., Yousof, Z., Munajat, I., Lee, N.A.A. and Zaki, N. (2011). Developmental dysplasia of hip screening using Ortolani and Barlow testing on breech delivered neonates. *Malays Orthopedic Journal*, **5**(3): 13–16.

UNICEF (n.d.) United Kingdom Baby Friendly Initiative. Available at: www.unicef.org.uk/babyfriendly/baby-friendly-resources/support-for-parents/tongue-tie.

Wilson, P., Hayes, E., Barber, A. and Lohr, J. (2016). Screening for spinal dysraphisms in newborns with sacral dimples. *Clinical Pediatrics*, **55**: 1064–70.

Clinical competence and professional responsibility

Christopher Lube and Tracey Jones

Introduction

This chapter explores clinical competence related to the neonatal infant physical examination (NIPE) and how this competence can be measured. A student guide to the NIPE could not be written without considering what defines clinical competence and what level a practitioner should aim to achieve. This is important not only for you as a student but also for those professionals working in the role as a NIPE practitioner. Public Health England (2016) emphasise the importance of this and highlight the professional responsibility to maintain competence once qualified as a NIPE practitioner. At this point in your learning you will no doubt have had to demonstrate competence in your work, be it academic or practical, but do you know how this was measured or what defines the level you are expected to achieve as a NIPE student? This chapter discusses competence and professional responsibility, including some of the teaching strategies that are being applied in learning institutions throughout the UK to help practitioners achieve clinical competence. A huge variation now exists in relation to current preparation of NIPE practitioners relating to academic accreditation, forms of assessment and the modes of content delivery. In nursing and midwifery education there is an ongoing transition from traditional teaching and learning to more self-directed and practice-based learning, and this is never more prevalent than in the education of the NIPE practitioner. Recognising the discussion in Chapter 2 related to the challenges linked to releasing practitioners from the workplace to attend classroom-based learning, new ways of teaching are being embraced.

THINK POINT

Take a moment to consider your NIPE course learning outcomes; how were you supported to achieve those outcomes?

What teaching methods were used to help you reach a point where you felt ready to perform your first NIPE in practice?

How the NIPE is taught

To become a NIPE practitioner requires midwives and neonatal nurses to attend a programme of formal education that includes a period of supervised practice, including assessment. As part of this learning you may have experienced a variety of teaching approaches to aid your learning, including simulation. The Patient Safety Strategy (World Health Organization [WHO], 2004), and acknowledgement of the complexity and multiple demands inherent in clinical nursing and midwifery, have driven the introduction of simulation for learning (Lejonqvist et al. 2016). Use of high-fidelity simulators offer learners effective and active learning (Murphy et al., 2011; Schmidt et al., 2011; Cook et al., 2013), and permits students to experience a variety of life-like situations in safe environments without jeopardising patient safety (Lejonqvist et al., 2016). You may have experienced simulation in your clinical environment or the university setting as part of the physical examination, or as a communication exercise. Whatever form of teaching was used the ultimate aim of simulation is to confirm and demonstrate that you have reached the level of knowledge and competence to safely commence a formative examination of the newborn. The number of formative and summative assessments will vary according to where you are completing your education because there is no set number for this, and studies show that there is no single teaching method that secures clinical competence and safe practice (Cook et al., 2013). Yearley et al. (2017) uncovered, in their study, that the number of NIPE examinations expected to be completed by NIPE pre-registration students to gain competence varied significantly, and some programmes had no set number. What this chapter will aim to do is to help you understand clinical competence, professional responsibility, accountability and clinical governance so that you might feel confident in your ability to move forward with your summative assessments. As practitioners governed by formal registration with the Nursing Midwifery Council, it is imperative that you fully understand your professional responsibility and the role that governance plays in healthcare safety. This chapter discusses the role of the NIPE practitioner in line with professional responsibility, making reference to the Nursing and Midwifery Council (NMC) Code for Nurses and Midwives (NMC, 2015).

> **THINK POINT**
>
> Contemplate for a moment what you understand by the term 'clinical governance' and why, as a NIPE practitioner, you need to be aware of it.

Smith (2012) defines clinical competence as motivation, assimilating knowledge into practice, experience, critical thinking skills, caring, communication and a supportive environment. Professionalism is considered to include confidence, safe practice and holistic care. All of these attributes and skills should be held by a NIPE practitioner.

Accountability in practice

It is expected that we are taught from an infant to be accountable for our actions and to take responsibility by being open and honest. For every healthcare professional, from the first exposure to clinical duties, we are required to be accountable for the activity, care and decisions that we make. Accountability is enshrined in a number of documents produced by professional and regulatory bodies (NMC, 2015a; Care Quality Commission, 2016) and by the UK government (Health and Social Care Act 2008). These place a legal requirement of accountability on the healthcare practitioner.

> **THINK POINT**
>
> Do you regularly review the NMC's Code as part of your reflective practice?

There are four parts to accountability – professional, ethical, employment and legal accountability – all of which play an essential role in ensuring that the care provided is safe and of a high quality, and in safeguarding the principle that healthcare professionals are held accountable.

By training to become a NIPE practitioner your current practice will change, in that you will be one of the professionals responsible for arguably the first important health screening that anyone undergoes. As such you have a duty to ensure that every NIPE you undertake is completed to the required standard and, where abnormalities are identified, that these are dealt with or escalated appropriately, following local policies and procedures. You are accountable for every element of the NIPE you will complete from start to finish, including your documentation.

Clinical governance

A principle that is closely related to personal accountability in clinical practice is clinical governance: a key framework that every healthcare organisation across the UK has established and implemented to ensure safe practice.

The development and introduction of clinical governance followed a number of high-profile 'failures' in the NHS, which included the Alder Hey Organ Retention Scandal (Redfern et al., 2001), the Bristol Heart Scandal (Kennedy, 2001) and the Shipman Inquiry (Smith, 2002, 2003), which led to a loss of public confidence in the safety of care being provided. Two key documents were produced by the government at the time: *The New NHS: Modern and Dependable* (Department of Health, 1997) and *A First Class Service: Quality in the NHS* (1998). These documents were designed to establish systems within the NHS to improve quality and safety, enabling trusts to gain assurances for themselves, patients/ public and the government. Governance over the years has moved forward, culminating in the introduction of the Health and Social Care Act 2008, making governance in the healthcare environment a legal requirement (Health and Social Care Act (Regulated Activity) 2014: Regulation 17). Clinical governance has been described in different ways, but always with the same theme: a system to ensure that care being provided, no matter by whom or where, is safe, and of high quality. Care provision has to be reviewed and monitored and, where issues, risks or complaints are identified, they are investigated and action taken to implement change and improvements. The goal is to ensure that the patient's experience of healthcare is one of safety and satisfaction.

THINK POINT

Consider for a moment how you would describe clinical governance to one of your more junior colleagues.

A number of definitions related to clinical governance have been produced since 1997. The main definition that has been used by many NHS organisations, produced by Scally and Donaldson (1998, p. 62), is:

> A framework through which organisations are accountable for continuously improving the quality of their services and safeguarding high standards of care by creating an environment in which excellence in clinical care will flourish.

In 2004, Chandra Vanu Som undertook a review of definitions of clinical governance since the one cited above in 1998 by Scally and Donaldson. Vanu Som found that none of the definitions reviewed captured the essence of clinical governance as defined by Scally and Donaldson in terms of the impact that clinical governance has on the implication for organisation-wide continuous quality improvement.

This can be linked to your everyday practice (Figure 9.1).

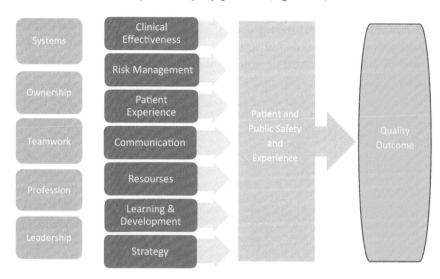

Figure 9.1
Elements of clinical governance (derived from Scally and Donaldson, 1998)

THINK POINT

Consider how accountability and clinical governance are linked.

For individual practitioners, clinical governance is about ensuring that you are competent in your role to provide high-quality safe care, which is in line with local policies and your employer's guidelines. The competencies or clinical outcomes that you have been given during your NIPE education will have been derived from aspects of governance and accountability.

THINK POINT

Consider you clinical practice documents: what level of competence do you have to achieve to pass your assessment?

The introduction of clinical governance systems is not limited to the UK. Countries worldwide have introduced systems to assess, monitor and review quality and safety of patient care. The need to identify and learn from incidents or poor quality of care is a worldwide priority. However, even though national and international systems and processes are developed to help improve this, it ultimately comes down to the individual practitioner to ensure that the care they are providing meets specified standards and one that the practitioner can take pride in as directed by the NMC's Code (NMC, 2015). Baston and Durward (2018) emphasise that expansion of practice such as that of a NIPE practitioner should be assumed in the full knowledge that employer support is in place because it will be the trust that will assume vicarious liability.

Accountability

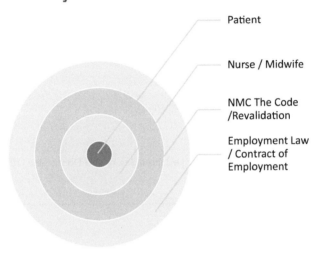

Patient

Nurse / Midwife

NMC The Code /Revalidation

Employment Law / Contract of Employment

Figure 9.2
Patterns of accountability (adapted from Walsh, 2000)

Professional accountability

Professional accountability is at the core of what nurses and midwives do every day and is also the core of the NMC's Code (NMC, 2015).

Clark (2000, p. 2), cited in Tilley and Watson (2004), defines professional accountability as

> a professional takes a decision or action not because someone has told him or her to do so, but because, having weighed up the alternatives and consequences in the light of the best available knowledge, he or she believes this it is right decision or action to take.

It is essential that as a NIPE practitioner any learning in relation to the care you are providing in this role benefits from safe care processes. Considering Benner levels of competency (Benner, 1984), you will be starting from a novice learner and must be clear to verbalise, with clinical mentors in practice, where your learning is at. As you start your clinical development in the NIPE as a novice learner, you must make your level of knowledge and experience explicit to those mentoring you in practice and negotiate the appropriate level of involvement you have in providing clinical care in relation to the NIPE.

Nurses and midwives are there to support and advocate for the patient, especially those who cannot advocate for themselves (Savage and Moore, 2004). This is a key role when undertaking the NIPE, especially as the patient is a newborn baby. Undertaking the NIPE practitioner role does not preclude use of all the other skills and experience gained as a nurse or midwife. Indeed, part of the value of undertaking this additional role as a neonatal nurse or midwife is that the holistic approach that underpins both professions' values is used. Taking a holistic approach to the role will enable practitioners to identify psychosocial or emotional issues that are not part of the physical examination. This is related directly to professional accountability by identifying how best to use the skills and knowledge you have to facilitate the best care for all patients as outlined in the Standards for Competence for Registered Nurses (NMC, 2010).

> ## THINK POINT
>
> Review your trust protocol related to the NIPE in practice and identify if it clearly outlines the professional accountability of the practitioner.

Employment accountability

Any contract of employment sets out a legal agreement between employer and employee as to their role and responsibility when undertaking the job they have been employed to undertake for payment. As a NIPE practitioner you have a contractual obligation to adhere to the guidance of your employing trust, and it is your responsibility to make yourself aware of your contractual obligation in relation to expanding any role that may be new or additional to that of your previous role.

It is essential as a NIPE practitioner that you fully understand your roles and responsibilities and ensure that you work within these. This is key when expanding as a professional and taking on additional responsibilities such as becoming a NIPE practitioner; this is also known as the 'scope of practice'. All nurses and midwives are expected to work within the 'scope of practice' assigned to the job they are employed to do. Working outside of this would mean that, if an incident occurred that led to a patient being harmed, the practitioner involved would not be covered by the organisation's indemnity insurance (Royal College of Nursing, 1998). Where a nurse or a midwife breaches one or more elements of their employment contract, this could lead to disciplinary action and dismissal from their employment.

> **THINK POINT**
>
> Read through your contract of employment and job description. Where are the limits that have been set by your employer? Do you know which NIPEs you are allowed to perform and which are deemed out of your scope of practice?

Ethical accountability

In the modern healthcare environment nurses and midwives confront ethical issues that require skills in ethical decision-making (Numminen and Leino-Kilpi, 2007). Understanding ethics and how this relates to accountability is just one element that nurses and midwives must consider. The main principles of ethics are beneficence and non-maleficence. Beneficence is the act of doing kindness and good for others. Nonmaleficence is the principle of not doing harm. So although beneficence is an action you take, nonmaleficence is when you avoid an action.

Legal accountability

Within UK society there are two types of law: civil and criminal. Each of these has its own set of processes and legal system structures. Every member of UK society is bound by these laws, and there is an expectation within society that nurses and midwives uphold these laws, in addition there is also an expectation from the MNC. As part of any nurse/midwives registration there is an expectation to report any infringements of the law to the NMC as part of your fitness to practice.

As a professional working in healthcare you have a duty of care to your patients, and this requires you to remain competent and offer a level of care determined by the Bolam test. As a NIPE practitioner you are performing a role previously dominated by paediatricians, so it is your responsibility to carry out that role with the same level of skill. You will be predominantly completing the NIPE on the term normal newborn; however, the medical team should be available if you highlight anything out of the normal that necessitates a review or you are concerned and need support.

Revalidation

As a midwife or nurse you have a duty to revalidate every 3 years (NMC, 2015b). This requires you to confirm that you have completed 450 hours of clinical practice and 35 hours of learning. As a NIPE practitioner you have an additional responsibility to ensure that you remain competent in this role, and it might be that your employer requires you to evidence this through a specific record. This might include attending theory updates or performing a specific number of examinations, which can be then used towards your revalidation process; it is your responsibility to be aware of your trust's requirement.

CLINICAL TIP

Consider keeping a diary or log of the dates that you complete NIPEs to evidence your practice.

Conclusion

The aim of this chapter was to provide an introduction to the area of clinical governance and accountability and how it applies to you as a NIPE practitioner. It is essential that all nurses and midwives understand that, as part of their registration with the NMC, they alone are responsible and accountable for ensuring their knowledge is up to date, they are competent, and working within their 'scope of practice' and within the law. It is also a key responsibility that when/if something goes wrong or a concern is identified, that you have a duty to escalate or report it.

Accountability and clinical governance are inextricably linked in everyday life for healthcare staff from ward to board. A nurse's duty of care binds them to providing the safest high-quality care, for which they are fully accountable at all times. To summarise there are four parts to accountability. and having an understanding of each enables you as a NIPE practitioner to offer safe, evidence-based, holistic and compassionate care to all of the babies whom you encounter when carrying out the NIPE.

References

Baston, H. and Durward, H. (2018). *Examination of the Newborn: A Practical Guide*, 3rd edn. London: Routledge.

Benner, P. (1984). *From Novice to Expert: Excellence and Power in Clinical Nursing Practice*. Menlo Park, CA: Addison-Wesley.

Care Quality Commission (2016). *The Fundamental Standards*. Available at: www.cqc.org.uk/what-we-do/how-we-do-our-job/fundamental-standards (accessed 25 April 2019).

Clark, J. (2000). Accountability in nursing. Second WHO Ministerial Conference on Nursing and Midwifery in Europe. Munich, 15–17 June.

Cook, D., Hamstra, S., Brydges, R., Zendejas, B., Szostek, J., Wang, A. et al. (2013). Comparative effectiveness of instructional design features in simulation based education: Systematic review and meta-analysis. *Medical Teaching*, **35**: 867–98.

Department of Health (1997). *The New NHS Modern and Dependable*. London, HSMO.

Department of Health (1998). *A First Class Service: Quality in the NHS*. London: Department of Health.

Kennedy, I. (2001). *Inquiry into the Management and Case of Children Receiving Complex Heart Surgery at the Bristol Royal Infirmary*. Norwich: HSMO.

Lejonqvist, G., Eriksson, K. and Meretoja, R. (2016). Evidence of clinical competence by simulation, a hermeneutical observational study. *Nurse Education Today*, **38**, 88–92.

Murphy, S., Hartigan, J., Walsh, N., Flynn, A. and O'Brien, S. (2011). Merging problem-based learning and simulation as an innovative pedagogy in nurse education. *Clinical Simulation Nursing*, **7**(4): e141–8.

Numminen, O.H. and Leino-Kilpi, H. (2007). Nursing students' ethical decision-making: a review of the literature. *Nurse Education Today*, **27**: 796–807.

Nursing and Midwifery Council (2010). *Standards for Competence for Registered Nurses*. London: NMC.

Nursing and Midwifery Council (2015a). *The Code: Professional standards of practice and behaviour for nurses and midwives*. London: NMC. Available at www.nmc.org.uk/globalassets/sitedocuments/nmc-publications/nmc-code.pdf (accessed 2 September 2018).

Nursing and Midwifery Council (2015b). *Revalidation. How to revalidate with the NMC*. London: NMC. Available at: http://revalidation.nmc.org.uk/ (accessed 2 September 2018).

Public Health England (2016). *Newborn and Infant Physical Examination Screening Programme Standards 2016/17*. Available at: www.gov.uk/government/uploads/system/uploads/attachment_data/file/524424/NIPE_Programme_Standards_2016_to_2017.pdf (accessed 20 April 2018).

Redfern, M., Keeling, J.W. and Powell, E. (2001). The Royal Liverpool Children's Inquiry: Summary and Recommendations, Available at: www.rlcinquiry.org.uk/download/sum.pdf.

Royal College of Nursing (1998). *Clinical Governance: An RCN Resource Guide*. London: RCN.

Savage, J. and Moor, L (2004). *Interpreting Accountability*. London: Royal College of Nursing.

Science Direct (2011). Licensing and Policies. Available at: www.sciencedirect.info/licensing.

Schmidt, H., Rotgans, J. and Yew, E., (2011). The process of problem-based learning: what works and why. *Medical Education*, **45**: 792–806.

Scally, G. and Donaldson, L.J. (1998). Clinical governance and the drive for quality improvement in the new NHS in England. *British Medical Journal*, **317**: 61–5.

Smith, J. (2002). *First Report: Death Disguised*. London: The Stationery Office.

Smith, J. (2003). Second Report: The Police Investigation of March 1998. Cmnd. 5853. London: The Stationery Office.

Smith, S. (2012). Nurse competence: A concept analysis. *International Journal of Nursing Knowledge*, **23**(3): 172–82.

Tilley, S. and Watson, R. (2004). *Accountability in Nursing and Midwifery*, 2nd edn. Oxford: Blackwell Publishing.

Vanu Som, C. (2004). Clinical governance: A fresh look at its definition. *Clinical Governance: An international Journal*, **9**(2): 87–90.

Walsh, M. (2000). *Nursing Frontiers: Accountability and Boundaries of Care*. London: Butterworth Heinemann.

World Health Organization (2004). *First Do No Harm, World Alliance for Patient Safety*. Washington, DC: WHO. Available at www.who.int/patientsafety/world alliance/en (accessed 2 September 2018).

Yearley, C., Rogers, C. and Jay, A. (2017). Including the newborn physical examination in the pre-registration midwifery curriculum: National survey. *British Journal of Midwifery*, **25**(1): 26–32.

The second examination

Tracey Jones

This chapter will help you to understand the need for the second examination completed between 6 and 8 weeks of age in the community setting.

This second examination is usually carried out by the general practitioner; however, more healthcare practices are employing advanced nurse practitioners to perform this screening examination. As with the neonatal infant physical examination (NIPE) carried out immediately after birth, this examination can be performed by any healthcare professional who has completed the NIPE qualification and is deemed competent. By developing an understanding of this examination you will be able to demonstrate a knowledge base and offer the family more information when you explain about this second screening test and alleviate any concerns that they might have. It is important that the parents are aware that all babies are offered this second test and that it usually coincides with the first immunisations. When you inform the parents that their infant requires a second examination, it might cause anxiety because they may presume that there is a concern and that something is abnormal with their child. However, this second examination is routine for all babies born in the UK. Information about the newborn and the 6- to 8-week-old infant physical examinations should be given to the parents during the antenatal period and again before the newborn examination is offered. It would be wise to check if your trust has any written information about these examinations because this can accompany your discussion, and offer the parents the opportunity to read further about the test once you have left.

It is important for practitioners carrying out the NIPE to fully understand what the 6- to 8-week check includes. It might be that you need to make a specific note about a finding in the child health booklet for the community practitioner to be aware of, such as a skin finding that you have referred but that needs to be monitored for growth and progression. If you consider the first examination, which highlights abnormalities that are detectable, within 72 hours of birth, the second check offers the opportunity for further identification of those abnormalities that may become detectable by age 6–8 weeks, during the second physical examination, and thereby reduce morbidity and mortality. These ages are recommended based on best practice and current evidence, and should facilitate a prompt referral for early clinical assessment.

> **THINK POINT**
>
> Consider you are carrying out a NIPE and you highlight one undescended testicle. You can feel the testis in the groin, so you do not need to make a referral. How will you explain this to the parents and how will the second check reassure them that they will see a practitioner again in the community.

The reason for the second examination is, first, that some conditions that can present will not be detected during the NIPE performed at age 72 hours or it might be that a condition that has been detected might resolve over the coming weeks. The second check is another opportunity to diagnose any abnormality, and offer reassurance and information to parents related to any abnormality previously diagnosed. If you consider specifically the cardiac chapter (Chapter 6B), which explains in more detail cardiac anomalies that may present after this first examination, by explaining this to the parents you offer more understanding of why the second examination is important to attend. Examination of the heart is very important because this may be the first time that a murmur will be audible. For example, if the infant has a ventricular septal defect (VSD), this may not have been apparent in the first 24 hours after birth.

In many cases the examination is now performed at 8 weeks to coincide with the first set of immunisations. This alleviates any unnecessary appointments because both the second NIPE and the set of first immunisations can be completed during one appointment. In addition to the physical check and immunisations, the examination should be used as an opportunity for the parents to raise any matters of concern. This is an opportunity for the baby's overall wellbeing to be assessed and a weight recorded.

> **THINK POINT**
>
> Consider what else could be discussed at this appointment.

This appointment is an ideal opportunity when feeding advice can be offered and referrals to other professionals can be made, should any other concerns be raised. It might be that the parents have a concern that they have not previously had the opportunity to discuss or something new might have occurred that they wish to have examined. The second consultation is an opportunity for parents to discuss any concerns related to their baby's tone or response. The community practitioner often works closely with the health visitor during this second check when there is an opportunity to discuss maternal factors such as how the mother is feeling and a discussion about contraception.

During this examination the eyes are examined for a second time so, if the infant has not reacted to visual stimulation, this can be explored further and referral can be made. The practitioner will ask the parents about the infant's responses and hearing can be discussed, asking again if the parents have any concerns. The hips will once again be examined during this check and, if any referrals have been missed, this is again an ideal chance to follow this up. If an abnormality was highlighted at the first NIPE then an ultrasound scan should have been performed. This can be discussed during this examination and followed up if any delays have occurred. As an NIPE practitioner it is beneficial for you to have an understanding of this second examination; this chapter has aimed to explain briefly some of the aspects of this examination to enable you to fully communicate and reassure the parents of further screening available.

As a NIPE practitioner, having an understanding of why this second examination should take place can help your confidence in discussions with parents and caregivers about the first examination.

Index

Printed and bound by CPI Group (UK) Ltd, Croydon, CR0 4YY

23/10/2024

01778226-0004